Chinese Medicine

Revealed

The Art of Long Life: A Complete Guide for Everyone

I0465675

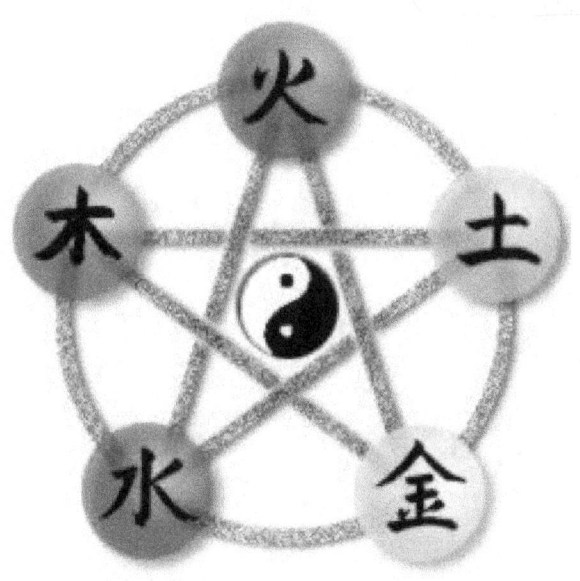

Tianren Wukong

SUMMARY

INTRODUCTION

1.1. Objectives and Structure of the Book

This manual is not intended to be a treatise on Chinese medicine or a comprehensive guide to Chinese Qigong. First and foremost, because Chinese medicine is so vast that it would require encyclopedias to cover it. The same applies to Qigong: it is said that there are 600 styles of Qigong.

Instead, this manual aims to provide a series of useful tools for maintaining or adopting a healthier lifestyle through the practice of simple but effective physical exercises, through paying attention to the messages our body sends us, and through greater awareness of ourselves and the world around us. There is no presumption of transforming our existence or our body, as many gurus try to do. "In 4 weeks. 10 minutes a day." And, I might add, maybe when you feel like it.

This manual reflects a desire to share a long journey of study and practice, where there may be some useful ideas and others that are less so, because we are not all the same and it is right that each of us should "assimilate" what most corresponds to our nature and leave out what does not belong to us. Today, perhaps with the passage of time, some ideas will re-emerge and become useful in another phase of our lives.

In this manual, you will find practices and explanations that are accessible and understandable to everyone, through the presentation of the "fundamentals" of Chinese medicine but, in accordance with the Pareto principle of 80% - 20% (i.e., that 20% of the information - quantitative data - contains 80% of the knowledge - qualitative data). Therefore, we will only cover the key principles without getting lost in the sophistication that may be of interest to specialists, but it is also true that in a holistic approach, we know that no two situations are ever identical, so it is good to investigate the key principles in order to get as close as possible to the truth. Furthermore, through a less specialized approach, I am confident that these ancient teachings can reach most people with the sole purpose of opening their minds to a culture that is fascinating but at the same time accessible to everyone.

1.2. The Importance of Well-being in the Modern Era

When I first became interested in Chinese medicine, I didn't know it, but I was about to embark on a journey of illness that I would only discover several years later, and many years later I would have to begin a therapy that will probably accompany me for the rest of my life. So, does Chinese medicine not work? Instead, I can say with certainty that my encounter with Chinese medicine and Eastern disciplines helped me open my mind to a spiritual path that has allowed me and continues to allow me to face this problem with more serenity and more presence in the "here and now."

It's an expression that is used and abused, but when I think about it, if I hadn't encountered this illness on my path, I would probably have maintained a level of stress, physical and mental fatigue, and professional performance anxiety that would have led me to psycho-physical exhaustion, or to some much more sudden and unexpected traumatic event.

Let's face it, our society, those of us born after the war, have seen the West gallop towards incredible levels of well-being, and to achieve them, increasingly demanding performances have been sought, the bar has been raised higher and higher, and so we are trying to achieve increasingly ambitious, complex, tiring... more inhuman results, but perhaps it would be more correct to say 'unnatural'. The night is not used to recover energy, alcohol is not used to extract essential oils, meat is not consumed only on special occasions, physical exertion is sought for a few hours a week for aesthetic reasons, while we dream of a job that involves no physical exertion and minimal mental exertion . All the values that have led humans to evolve over the millennia and build an advanced civilization are now being overturned, and with them, our mental and physical well-being. Nature has always provided us with all the resources we need to live well, eat perfectly, and live peacefully until the age of 80—many Greek and Roman philosophers reached this age without any problems—but now we need to supplement our diet with vitamins, minerals, elements to help us sleep, or to keep us awake, or to stop us worrying, or to digest something that has been eaten for thousands of generations: this simply means that we have lost our balance, we have lost innate resources or those present in nature because, in order to be successful, we have had to sacrifice something: time to rest, time to eat well, time to devote to our loved ones, time to watch a sunrise or sunset. Yet in our hearts we know what those values or those little moments are that make a day, or a life, special. We are on the merry-go-round, we cannot get off, but when we have the opportunity, we recognize when it is time to stop and fully savor the "here and now"... we could learn to do without it and want to give a new direction to our hectic journey.

1.3. Illness

In imperial China, doctors were paid when people were healthy and received no compensation when they fell ill. Their work was therefore one of prevention and education, because treating the sick would have been extraordinary, unpaid work, and for this reason they had to trust in the patient's quick recovery.

This is exactly the opposite of what happens today: we only go to the doctor when we are not well, when illness has set in, and they prescribe medication or increasingly expensive check-ups to investigate where we have 'gone wrong'. The point is that we have made a mistake because no one has given us the instructions for our machine. Perhaps we made a mistake when we forgot about ourselves until illness came knocking at our door, or an energy or mental health problem. In short: as long as everything is fine, no one is interested in the only body we have. Then, when something goes wrong, a mechanism is triggered that is often a source of further stress, financial hardship (let's not deny it, getting healthcare has become a privilege), and immense waste of time (we will come back to this point at the end). Yet all we needed to do was oil the gears along the way. Didn't anyone tell us? False, someone is trying , but we always look for the easiest way out: better to stuff ourselves with drugs than to stop for two or three days to rest, hydrate, and let the flu pass; better to show that a slight fever can't stop me and I can continue to produce (for whom?) than to rest at home and not infect anyone, recover my energy more completely without risking a relapse; better to take anti-inflammatories for that muscle discomfort than to understand the reason for it and maybe do some corrective exercises... The examples are endless, and the collapse of the public health system should make us reflect on the need to oil our gears rather than turn to the mechanic when a part breaks. Because maybe the part is expensive and takes too many months of suffering, limitations, and discomfort to get.

If, on the other hand, we take a less rational approach, we should remember when we have been ill. Perhaps in a year we catch the flu and spend the most memorable 5-7 days of the last 365. Is this possible? Yes, because illness is a nuisance, a discomfort, it deprives us of time to live. So we should be diligent and try to prevent illness from affecting us. It is also true that not everyone is 'strong' enough by nature to avoid illness. Everyone is susceptible. Many are affected, few are not. But the difference is that if a person is healthy, they will be affected, but the course of the illness will be short and leave no lasting effects.

Today's doctors should give us these instructions: strengthen your body to face illness as a winner, but this is not the case, so it is up to us to take action to achieve this result and try to see the doctor as little as possible. And take responsibility for our health.

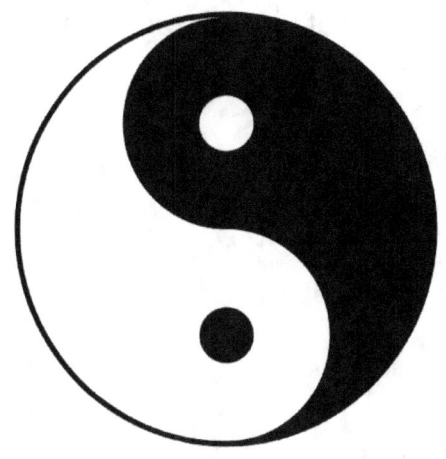

The Tao, composed of Yin (dark part) and Yang (light part)

"Every long journey begins with a single step" - Laozi

2. BASIC PRINCIPLES OF CHINESE MEDICINE

2.1. Origins and Evolution of Chinese Medicine

Chinese medicine has a thousand-year history and has developed into five main strands:

1.   Acupuncture and moxibustion

2.   Massage

3.   Exercise (or Qigong)

4.   Diet

5.   Herbal medicine

Therefore, a good Chinese doctor knows all these techniques, even if they tend to specialize in one or two of them. Let's say that each of them has characteristics that may be suitable for one individual and perhaps less so for another.

Massage, for example, requires a good ability on the part of the practitioner to move their own Qi and that of the recipient, creating harmony and restoring balance to the recipient's Qi. Input is received from outside.

Acupuncture and moxibustion have a dynamic and warming function, but there is less interaction with the recipient. Acupuncture is practiced by applying needles to specific points (called acupoints) that represent energy "nodes" and follow defined paths called meridians. Moxibustion works on the same points but uses a tool that produces heat (moxa, which is mugwort wool in the form of balls or cigars to be placed near the points) and also helps to combat cold symptoms. Input is received from outside.

Dietetics requires a good knowledge of physiology according to Chinese medicine and an assessment of the individual to provide the right nutrition (right in terms of quality and quantity). Anyone can study this in depth to eat properly, but it requires an in-depth study of the principles of Chinese medicine, physiology, and the energy dynamics of food, which is already a very demanding task for a non-professional. Input is received from outside.

Herbal medicine is the equivalent of Western pharmacopoeia and is certainly the most complex and articulated. In China, it represented the final stage of Chinese medical studies, requiring up to 20 years of practice before one could call oneself an herbalist. Herbal medicine has a much more intense effect than dietetics; it can be compared to acupuncture in relation to massage. Input is received from outside.

Finally, Qigong requires knowledge of the body and good proprioception on the part of the practitioner. It is certainly a practice that Chinese medicine doctors must know and practice because it serves to rebalance, regenerate, and reorganize their energies. The Chinese do not judge by appearance, but if they had to rely on a doctor who appeared to be overweight or with obvious pathologies, they would be wary because those who do not take care of themselves cannot be trusted to take care of others. Clothes do not make the man, of course, but it is discipline that characterizes Eastern practices, and this should already make us understand that the difference between the two cultural approaches diverges from the outset, from those who must set a good example (and I avoid applying this reasoning to other areas because the defeat of the Western world would be immediate and without possibility of redemption). Input is received from both inside and outside.

2.2 Philosophy and methodology

The earliest written records of medical practices date back more than 4,000 years, and it is not possible to date the birth of one practice before another with certainty, but Qigong is probably the oldest practice as it derives from shamanic dances, even before the codification of points and meridians (which characterize acupuncture, moxibustion, and massage). Over the centuries, various techniques developed, partly depending on the geographical location of the various scholars. The fact that China is the size of a continent and has every possible climate imaginable has allowed for the development of a variety of schools and 'styles' in every discipline: the cuisine of the north is different from that of the south, as are the styles of Kung Fu, and even the physical appearance of the Chinese, who are tall in the north and smaller in the south (and therefore also developed styles of Kung Fu more suited to their characteristics). Certainly, in the south, moxa was studied and developed to a much more limited extent than in the north or in Tibet. The variety and continuous exchange of information has therefore allowed for the creation of many schools of thought and practice (it is said that there are 600 styles of Qigong in China!) and certainly, the empirical approach has ensured that each of these practices, if they have survived millennia, wars, and pandemics, are effective. To conclude and understand the importance of Chinese medicine, consider that during Mao's Chinese Cultural Revolution, he tried to eliminate everything that was traditional, a product of ancient culture, to allow China to enter the modern world. However, during the 1950s, an encephalitis pandemic broke out that allopathic medicine was unable to contain. Mao then allowed the use of acupuncture, and the pandemic was controlled and eradicated. This led to a process of recovery and modernization of medicine, which is now referred to as traditional Chinese medicine, but which in reality has a more scientific and engineering-based approach. Ancient Chinese medicine, on the other hand, is defined as Classical Medicine, and the only texts that survived the cultural purge were found in Korea and Japan, so paradoxically, it is easier to find a doctor who practices classical Chinese medicine in Japan than in China. But these aspects are of little importance to our discussion.

Undoubtedly, Chinese medicine developed hand in hand with the three main philosophies of ancient China: Taoism, Confucianism, and Buddhism. We refer to philosophy and not, improperly, religion, as these three schools of thought arose and developed independently of religion. It is true that both Taoism and Buddhism developed a religious aspect, but it is very different from the concept we have in the West. Therefore, we will discuss three philosophies— —which originated around the 7th century BC and have different principles that can be summarized as follows:

- Taoism and the integration of the individual with the cosmos (and nature in general)

- Buddhism and the overcoming of suffering through love, compassion, and kindness

- Confucianism and ethics.

Undoubtedly, in classical Chinese medicine schools, Taoism is the school of thought that has most influenced the study and practice of the various disciplines. It has proven to be the most organized, structured, and consistent with the basic principles of this philosophy. Furthermore, by understanding the principles of Taoism, without delving too deeply into the studies, we can acquire sufficient tools to operate independently in our quest for health.

2.3. The Holistic Approach to Health

If you are not a holistic practitioner, do you know what 'holistic' means? Very often, people translate 'holistic' as 'new age', 'hippies', 'peace and love' or similar concepts. No! Holistic has ancient origins, from the Greek 'olos', meaning 'whole, entire', and refers to an approach that takes into account the individual as a whole: body, mind and spirit, emotions, feelings, organs, fluids, functions, age, work, living environment, season, date of birth, physiognomy...

Chinese medicine is certainly one of the types of medicine that takes into account many factors characterizing the individual in order to have as many pieces of information as possible to make a complete diagnosis. Let's use the metaphor of a jigsaw puzzle. Let's assume that making a diagnosis and understanding the causes of an individual's ailments based on their type is a graphic representation and that it takes the form of a jigsaw puzzle. The more information we gather and combine, the more pieces we will have in our puzzle and the better we will be able to understand what is represented. Perhaps with 80 pieces out of a 100-piece puzzle, it will be quite simple. On the other hand, a diagnostic approach that attempts to trace the pathology exclusively from the symptoms is like reducing the number of pieces to ten, twenty at most. This is not a criticism, but rather a statement of fact. Don't believe it? Then ask yourself how many times your doctor has asked you:

- Date of birth (to find out the astrological element of when you were born)

- Did they examine your tongue?

- He palpated your wrists

-        He asked you questions about whether you feel cold or hot, how you sleep, if you wake up at night and at what time, and what your urine and stools are like

-        Did he ask you what kind of dreams you have?

-        Did they ask you if there are times of day when you feel differently than usual: cold, hot, tired?

-        If you have cold knees, a cold abdomen, a cold lower back, a cold neck...

-        He looked at your fingernails

These are just some of the factors that Chinese medicine takes into consideration, but there are many others. And as in the example of the puzzle, the need for a lot of information is necessary because sometimes pieces seem to fit in one position but then they don't fit perfectly with the adjacent pieces. This is because there can be several causes that generate a disorder, but one can never assume that there is a cause and effect. Certain causes can generate complex situations that then materialize in effects that are not immediately attributable to the first factor. This is why a frame is built within a frame, within a frame: to be almost certain of having identified the diagnosis.

This methodical approach stems from the fact that in ancient China, the emperor's physician was killed if the emperor fell ill, so he had to be flawless. Normal doctors, on the other hand, were paid when their patients were well. Sick people were a great nuisance because they took up a lot of the doctor's time, as he had to find the cause of the illness, find a remedy, try it out, check its effectiveness... so it was a drain on resources and time. And if the doctor wanted to eat, he had to have healthy patients, so he had to be good and effective. And if he wasn't good, he would have had many sick patients who would have reported him as an incompetent doctor, and he would have risked losing his patients.

Don't you think that things are diametrically opposed in our society?

No one wants to replace their doctor or specialist, but it is useful to learn to listen to ourselves, to feel ourselves and to tune in to our inner voice, which can help us understand where we could do better to improve our health, whether it be in terms of diet, lifestyle, physical activity or any other insight that is useful for ourselves.

3. DYNAMIC DUALISM: YIN AND YANG

3.1 Polarity as a universal law

One of the most widely known symbols associated with Chinese medicine, Chinese culture, martial arts, and everything related to the concept of "Zen" is the symbol of the Tao, or Taijitu. It is a circle composed of two small fish: one white and one black (originally the colors were black and red, and later we will understand why).

To understand the approach of Chinese practices, it is necessary to grasp this fundamental principle because it is the basis of the balances and choices we face every day. Understanding it is essential for a practice that seeks perfect balance. This does not mean 'in medio stat virtus', whereby we must try to conform to the norm. The theory of yin and yang tells us that sometimes it is necessary to add yin, remove yang... or in any case find the right combination to achieve our balance: based on who we are, constitutionally, mentally, spiritually, and based on the path we have taken—work, family, projects...

Yin: represents the dark part of the symbol and identifies the feminine, the cold, stillness, the north, matter.

Yang: represents the light part of the symbol and identifies the masculine, heat, dynamism, the south, energy.

As can be seen in the symbol, in each area there is a small dot of the opposite element. This is because there is always a 'seed' of the opposite element from which one of the elements is generated. There is never an absolute condition because if there were 100% Yin, there would be death (only matter, cold and without movement... does that remind you of anything?), while 100% Yang would mean... death (only energy, volatility, spirit...).

We are used to thinking in a dualistic way, and I noticed this while studying Chinese medicine when my friends asked me if Yin was good or bad, if they were Yin or Yang, and there was no answer, nor will there ever be. There is no good or bad, you are not one or the other, but you are a little bit of both, perhaps with a prevalence, a tendency, but you have to learn about yin and yang and get to know yourself so that you don't get scared or worried when, for whatever reason (illness, stress, accidents...), the balance within us (whether physical or mental).

So let's think of Yin as fuel and Yang as the flame: we must always have a supply of fuel and th , otherwise the flame will burn out at a certain point. This teaches us that there are rhythms to be respected in our existence, which are repeated periodically throughout the seasons and throughout the day. Sleep and rest allow us to restore Yin (the phase in which the parasympathetic system is activated), which will gradually be converted into Yang during the day to allow us to carry out essential daily activities.

I repeat: this manual is not intended to be a manual of Chinese medicine or Chinese medical physiology: it aims to offer everyone a series of fundamental concepts and principles that are useful for taking a different approach to our lives, caring for our bodies, and so on. It is simplified and summarized as much as possible for reasons of usefulness. If you wish to explore the concepts and functional principles of Chinese medicine in greater depth, please refer to more comprehensive and specific treatises.

It is important to understand that there is no Yin and Yang, but rather a Yin/Yang relationship: every phenomenon, every situation, every reality must be "measured" in relation to another. Where there is life, there cannot be absolute Yin or Yang. For example: water is more Yin than fire, but more Yang than ice. This is an extreme but simple example to understand how to approach this type of assessment. The shoulders are more Yang than the knees (because they are higher up), and even more Yang than the feet. But the chest will be more Yin than the shoulder blades, even though they are at the same height, because the front of the body is conventionally Yin while the back is Yang.

Phenomena and situations are permeated by a quantity of Yin and a quantity of Yang, which varies and relates to the outside world: imagine pouring drops of ink into clear water. The more drops we pour, the darker the water becomes. The relationship between Yin and Yang is this increasing change in intensity of one element compared to another.

If we think about it, this rhythm follows the trend of the percentage of fluids in our body:

we are born 80% water and gradually dry out to around 60%. So from a greater Yin to a reduction of the same, and the more Yin there is, the more Yang can manifest itself, so in youth, we are energetic and dynamic, and as Yin is consumed, Yang also becomes more contained. The same applies to annual rhythms, whereby we are more inclined to be active in summer and more conservative in the colder seasons (winter is Yin and summer is Yang). During the day, as we have already seen, wakefulness is the Yang phase and rest is the Yin phase.

3.2. The Balance of Yin and Yang in the Human Body

There is a saying: "He who hesitates is lost," which is true, but if we don't stop, we burn out.

Therefore, the theory of Yin and Yang represents the first form of balance that we should apply, learning to know ourselves, learning to plan our lives, in order to face every moment with the best possible energy level (Yin fuel + Yang flame). In fact, certain activities are recommended at certain times of the day rather than others. For example, it would be ideal to do more intense physical activity in the morning, when we have restored our fuel level to its maximum, while in the evening it would be more appropriate to do more "quiet" activities (meditation, Qigong, Yoga, pranayama...) both because there may be little fuel left (even though in truth the vast majority of work activities involve low energy expenditure), and because it is good not to rekindle the flame before going to rest.

Balance therefore consists not in maintaining a 50% level of Yin and Yang, but in knowing how to dose one's energies so as not to exhaust one or the other, as well as knowing how to organize one's time in such a way as to be able to restore one's energies correctly and carry out activities (work and non-work) in such a way as not to compromise one or the other (r vice versa). (for example, compensating for sedentary work with suitable physical activity), eating in such a way as to balance an overly yang nature with yin foods, rather than according to the season...

Below are some of the situations that can lead to a disharmony between Yin and Yang.

1) An excess of Yang (perhaps due to external causes such as heatstroke or an overly warming diet) consumes Yin and, over time, compromises fluids. If Yang remains in excess (no cold compresses are applied or no change is made to the diet), Yang will always remain in excess and fluids will be consumed more and more (this condition generally affects the blood).

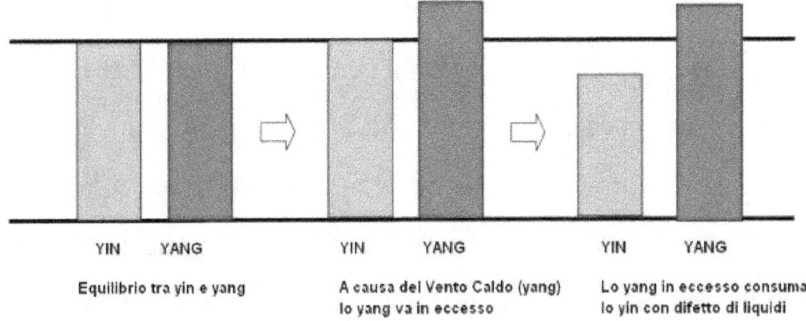

YIN   YANG   YIN   YANG   YIN   YANG

Equilibrio tra yin e yang   A causa del Vento Caldo (yang)   Lo yang in eccesso consuma
lo yang va in eccesso   lo yin con difetto di liquidi

2)   An excess of Yin (for example, due to exposure to cold or the ingestion of cold foods that block the Yang in the stomach) causes a weakening of Yang. The persistence of this situation leads to cold extremities, lower back pain, and joint pain. Cold enters through the feet, so it is good to warm them and keep them warm.

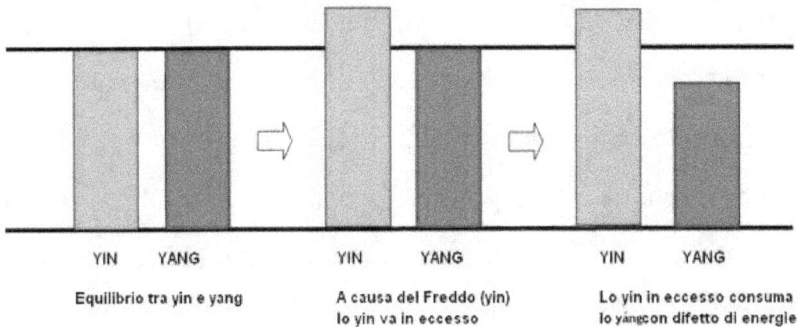

YIN   YANG   YIN   YANG   YIN   YANG

Equilibrio tra yin e yang   A causa del Freddo (yin)   Lo yin in eccesso consuma
lo yin va in eccesso   lo yangcon difetto di energie

3)   A relative Yang deficiency (compared to the balance line, which is a subjective and personal condition for which there is no objective value valid for all individuals) has effects similar to an excess of Yin (coldness, sluggishness) but over time, without the contribution of Yang, which cannot transform Yin, the condition of Yin will also worsen and you may feel that you are in Yin/Yang balance but in fact you have lost something in terms of energy, vitality, food assimilation...

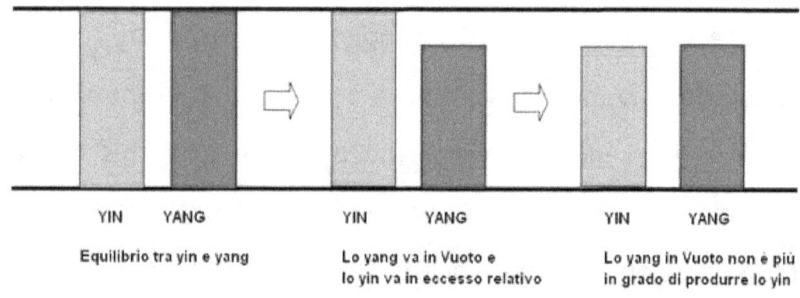

YIN   YANG   YIN   YANG   YIN   YANG

Equilibrio tra yin e yang   Lo yang va in Vuoto e   Lo yang in Vuoto non è più
                              lo yin va in eccesso relativo   in grado di produrre lo yin

4)   A relative Yin deficiency (compared to the balance line) has similar effects to Yang excess, but it is a false heat, so, for example, there is a lack of sweating. over time, without the contribution of Yin (which is the root of Yang), Yang will also be reduced and, as in the previous scenario, you will feel Yin/Yang balanced but in fact you will have lost something in terms of energy, vitality, food assimilation...

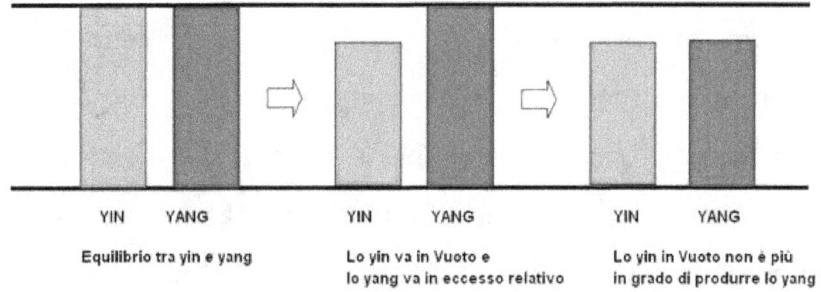

YIN   YANG   YIN   YANG   YIN   YANG

Equilibrio tra yin e yang   **Lo yin va in Vuoto e**   **Lo yin in Vuoto non è più**
                                     lo yang va in eccesso relativo   **in grado di produrre lo yang**

3.3. Restoring Harmony between Yin and Yang

Chinese medicine does not in any way seek to fix the individual at the midpoint because this is impossible. If we consider that one of the classic Chinese philosophical works is the I Ching - The Book of Changes: it is therefore expected that everything is in constant evolution and mutation, there is no idea of 'fixing' an individual in a state of balance because a change in external temperature, an overly abundant meal, or an excessively tiring day is enough to shift this balance. The individual, therefore, must have the tools to understand these changes, feel them, and have a series of remedies that can bring them as close as possible to equilibrium, but also in relation to the future. Let's think about when, having to undertake a long and tiring journey, we force ourselves to go to bed early the night before. A long and tiring day involves the consumption of Yang and, after a certain time, the consumption of Yin. So we try to stock up on Yin (hours of sleep). This example illustrates Yin/Yang physiology, but it is clear that it is innate in us, when common sense emerges, an approach that tends to seek a balance between activity and rest, but which translates biologically into the activity of the sympathetic (Yang) and parasympathetic (Yin) systems, energy consumption, and the restoration of our resources.

When we exhaust Yang, we can choose to stop and restore it or continue what we are doing, thus beginning to consume Yin. If we think of prolonged physical activity (or prolonged work, even if not necessarily physically demanding), after a certain number of hours we will exhaust Yang (which we should call Yang Qi), for which we will have to draw on Yin, convert it into Yang, and move forward. Example: going for a long run without preparing properly or without supplementing with the right foods during the run. After a certain point, our body will start to 'consume' muscles (Yin), and physical trauma such as strains or tears may occur... and then recovery times are longer than a long restorative sleep or recovery with half a day of rest.

Yang is a fast energy, it recovers in a few hours. Yin is more structural, therefore slow to regenerate (like a wound that needs to heal), and its excessive consumption can lead to long recovery times.

So the balance lies in knowing our own limits and, depending on what we have to do, organizing our resources so that we do not end up in a state of excessive stress where returning to balance requires a long time or external intervention.

Question: but what if we find ourselves in a situation where we have also exhausted our Yin... what happens then? Our body draws energy from Jing, the most Yin substance in our body. However, we will talk about this later in . For now, it is important to understand how this polarity of dynamism/rest, consumption/replenishment, must be managed correctly, judiciously, perhaps by testing our limits, because no two individuals have the same energy consumption levels, knowing full well that maximum well-being does not lie in maximum performance or maximum rest, but rather in the situation of an individual who has the maximum potential for performance: they may or may not express it, but the athlete is in their best condition before bending down to position themselves on the starting blocks: at the peak of their energy, their mind is clear of thoughts but perceives any input from the outside as if it were a sword stroke and feels capable of flying. That 'status', that condition, is the goal to be achieved when we face each day, each challenge, each activity, oscillating between different Yin/Yang energy levels and finding our dynamic balance. Because static balance gets us nowhere on our journey.

A safe, effective remedy with no contraindications is to drink hot or warm beverages, definitely in the morning but also recommended before meals (in many countries, meals begin with hot broth) because it helps the stomach (which is Yang and has a Yang function, so if you give it a hot drink = Yang, you help its digestive function). In addition, a hot drink contains Yin (water) and Yang (heat energy), so it can help and support the person if they are in the conditions highlighted in the previous graphs in cases 3 and 4. Finally, a hot drink has a muscle-relaxing effect, so at the end of the day it also helps to relieve muscle and tendon tension.

Yang exercise: greeting spring.

As soon as we wake up, our Yang begins to circulate again, so it is good to go with the flow and let it flow throughout the body. This exercise, which mainly stretches and relaxes the muscles of the back and legs, facilitates the flow of Yang in the Tai Yang meridian, where our Qi begins to flow when we open our eyes. Essentially, we stretch our muscles and move our joints as if we were stretching a water pipe, to allow the liquid (in this case Qi - energy) to flow better inside it.

Movement 1) Rotate your shoulders backward and rise onto your toes while inhaling. Once the rotation is complete, return your weight to your whole foot and, exhaling slowly, wrap your back (head, shoulders, chest, abdomen) around your hands as you descend toward your feet, massaging the lateral fascia of your legs. Finish exhaling by touching your feet and massaging the inside of your legs. Rise up again, inhaling and unrolling your back (abdomen, chest, shoulders, and head is the last part to straighten), rise up onto your toes, rotate your shoulders, and start again. Repeat 9 times.

Movement 2) Shake your body, bending your knees repeatedly and suddenly, as if you were a sack of beans, and try to move everything towards your feet. Keep your spine and head straight, without bending or swaying; it is the rest of your body that should be vibrating. Do this for at least 30 seconds to a minute. It helps to relieve tension in the shoulders.

Movement 3) Starting with my right hand, I pretend to pick up a bucket in front of me and lift it in front of my left knee, making a wide rotation of my right shoulder. My right foot is rotated, resting only on the tip, and my right knee touches my left knee. My back is straight and I look forward, so my spine is slightly twisted. Returning to the front, I perform the same movement with my left hand, picking up the bucket and lifting it in front of my right knee. 9 times on each side. Breathe freely.

This exercise helps to stretch and activate all the posterior muscles (from the calves to the thighs, buttocks, and the entire dorsal and cervical area). The shaking movements relieve tension or slight contractures, and the third movement activates the helical movement (characteristic of tai chi and Chinese martial arts) to twist the muscles and, above all, the vertebra I column. In fact, exercises that involve twisting the torso 'wash the marrow', i.e. they cleanse the marrow and improve the production of white and red blood cells, thus providing essential support for the immune system.

Yin exercise: Heron walk.

This exercise is very simple. In the different styles of Qigong, there are many walks, some more complex than others. Yin is the essential matter, water, nourishment, it does not need complexity or artificial elements: these will be introduced by adding Yang elements, moving on to wood and fire.

It is recommended to start by standing with your feet together and upright for at least 5 breaths. If you have time, it is recommended to stay in this position for 2 minutes. To harmonize and calm your breathing, bringing it down below your navel, push your head upwards, stretch your spine, relax your shoulders, unhook your knees, feel the weight on the soles of your feet, mainly on your heels and the outer part (the bony part, the arch of the foot should not bear any weight). Then decide to lift one foot and bring the knee up to hip height, creating a 90-degree angle. At the same time, raise your hands (fingers not clenched but apart) sideways to about ear height. Your elbows should be pointing towards your lower abdomen and slightly bent, with your wrists relaxed. As you raise your legs and arms, inhale slowly, bringing the air below your navel, but without exaggerating the protrusion of your belly. Then move on to the exhalation phase, even slower, with your hands descending like a flapping of wings, so that your elbows and wrists bend slightly, reaching hip height. The foot descends, taking a step that is not too long, and the sole of the foot lands horizontally, without the heel or forefoot touching first. The whole sole at the same time. To facilitate the step, you may also need to bend the knee of the supporting leg slightly, as if it were a piston. Then start again with the other leg, inhaling and raising your arms. Ideally, you should walk in a fairly wide circle (about twenty steps). Your gaze should be on the horizon and never towards the ground or the sky, your shoulders should always be relaxed, and you should feel your arms as if they were light wings lifted by the air you breathe into your lungs when you inhale. Once I have finished walking, I return to the starting position and focus my attention on the weight on my heels and the upward thrust from my heels, supporting my head as it floats in the air. The slowness and depth of my breathing determine how much I can charge my Yin.

Walking, however simple it may seem, provides numerous stimuli: first of all, balance, which is achieved thanks to complete proprioception from how the foot is placed, how weight is carried on it, the mobility of the ankles and knees, the emptying of the hips, the holding of the abdomen, the relaxation of the breath, and the head thrown back toward the sky. This is the 'static' part, then there is the dynamic part, with the transition from the yang leg (the one on which the weight is carried) to the yin leg (the one that is raised) and which becomes yang in the next step. The legs alternate, yin and yang, but the hips always remain empty, the knees and ankles flexible and free, the breathing relaxed and the head held high.

4 – PRINCIPLES: THE 5 MOVEMENTS

4.1 Nature as a guide

Over the course of approximately 5,000 years of codified Chinese medicine, there have been many schools and theories. In addition to theories based on Yin and Yang, another fundamental strand is that of the 5 elements.

The theory of the 5 elements also pervades all levels of thought, physiology, and cosmology in Chinese culture, allowing for a vast interpretation and application of phenomena relating to one element rather than another.

The five elements—or more correctly, movements—are: earth, metal, water, wood, and fire. We start with the natural elements and then interpret how phenomena manifest themselves and how relationships occur. For this reason, they should actually be defined as 'movements' – unlike our method of classification into elements – but in the end, many Western texts refer to them as elements. It can be misleading to think of them as static rather than dynamic factors that generate relationships between the elements (which do interact).

To explain its nature, in fact, an indication is given of how Qi manifests itself in these movements: water descends, fire rises, wood expands ( ), metal contracts, earth transforms and stabilizes. But what do these movements do? What are they?

According to Chinese medicine, they are manifestations of Qi based on their dynamics, and each organ or viscera is characterized by one of them. Wood is associated with the liver and gallbladder, fire with the heart, small intestine, pericardium, and triple heater, earth with the stomach and spleen/pancreas, metal with the lungs and large intestine, and finally water with the kidneys and urinary bladder.

Therefore, each organ or viscera has its own characteristic dynamics, which are inhibited or exacerbated in pathological cases. A typical example is wood, where excessive movement will result in excess Yang and can lead to outbursts of anger, rage, etc. If, on the other hand, the dynamism of wood and vegetative growth is stopped, there will be liver stasis with symptoms of repressed anger rather than indecision.

A healthy person will have organs with the right dynamism according to the elements. In addition, each person will have a characterizing element from which a typical character will result, for example

wood: determination

fire: joy and creativity

earth: transformation

metal: introspection

water: regeneration

On the other hand, if an element is particularly distressed, pathological conditions may occur:

wood: indecision or anger

fire: excitement or confusion

earth: brooding

metal: sadness

water: fear.

4.2 Levels

Shifting our attention to the concept of levels, according to Chinese medicine, each individual is made up of different "layers," from the densest (bones, muscles, organs) to the most "subtle" (emotions, feelings, senses). Every movement has an effect on all layers, therefore simultaneously on both organs and emotions.

Therefore, if there is a problem at the 'wood' level, problems with liver or gallbladder function may arise, or psychological problems such as indecision or anger. There may also be other side effects, such as vision problems (the liver opens into the eyes), brittle nails, or frequent cramps. In short, every movement has its own possible pathological manifestation on these different levels. We could simplify the division of an individual's levels into three: physical, emotional, and spiritual, to use a more "Western" classification, but this would not be correct as the levels differ in the density of Qi. Everything is Qi, this is the principle, only the density of Qi changes, so the Qi of the wood movement manifests itself, where it is denser, in the liver, in the eyes, in sharpness of vision, in anger or determination, up to the Hun, or the spiritual manifestation that resides in the liver. And so on with all the elements. So when we talk about the energy of wood, the lodge of wood, etc., we must consider that its nature is univocal but its manifestation is manifold according to the density of the Qi that represents it.

From a physical point of view, there are some typical combinations that can be useful in identifying the presence of problems in one element rather than another, as they are actually visible:

wood: eye/sight, nails, tendons,

fire: taste, blood, and capillaries

earth: touch, complexion

metal: smell, skin

water: hearing, hair, teeth.

4.3 Polarity in movements

If we were to think in terms of Yin and Yang in order to integrate the principles outlined in the previous chapter on Yin and Yang with the principles of the 5 movements, we would have fire as the most Yang movement and water as the most Yin, with the other movements being a transition with increasing Yang (wood) or increasing Yin (metal), all with an intermediate phase for each transition given by earth, which is transformation. It is the intermediate phase par excellence; in fact, in some texts, it is not represented in one of the positions of a pentagon, as is usually found in Chinese medicine manuals, but is placed at the center of a cross. Understanding that there is a Yin/Yang dynamic between the movements is necessary to interpret change and trends, but also to understand what kind of action should be taken to correct a pathological attitude. In fact, a Yang tendency in wood (anger) or fire (excitement) will be tempered with a Yin-type intervention (rest, meditation, sedation).

Law of generation

Going deeper into the theory of the 5 movements, it is important to know that they have a mother/child relationship: wood is the mother of fire, which is the mother of earth, which is the mother of metal, which is the mother of water, which in turn is the mother of wood. Do we remember this? Wood is obtained from plants, which can be burned, and once completely burned, it becomes ash (earth), which, once compacted and condensed, becomes metal, and from this, water is generated, which hydrates and nourishes plants, and the cycle starts again.

Therefore, as in the parental relationship, if one movement is deficient, the child will in turn be deficient because it has not been sufficiently nourished by the mother. For this reason, there is no privileged movement/organ: if one of them is depleted, it will affect the next one, which will in turn affect the one after that. So it is obvious that if one movement is neglected, everyone will ultimately pay the consequences. Furthermore, it is worth pointing out at this point that the mother-child relationship, in terms of organ energy, is subject to the principles of Yin and Yang. This is because the organs (considered full and with a specific function in the physiology of the body) are Yin in nature, while the viscera (empty and with a transport function) are Yang in nature.

Movement	Yin	Yang
Wood	Liver	Gallbladder

Fire	Heart	Small intestine
	Pericardium	Triple heater
Earth	Spleen / Pancreas	Stomach
Metal	Lungs	Large intestine
Water	Kidney	Urinary bladder

Therefore, if the mother is a Yin organ and is deficient, she will not sufficiently nourish her Yin child. But at the same time, within the same element, a weakness of the Yin organ could lead to an "excess" of the corresponding Yang viscera.

This brings us back to the basic concept that the goal of Chinese medicine and Chinese medical practices is to restore balance where it has been disrupted by an excess or deficiency of movement or its corresponding opposite polarity.

Law of control

The other law that relates movements is the law of control, which is called 'grandfather-grandson', where a movement has a controlling action on the subsequent movement of the son, thus:

Wood controls earth, fire controls metal, earth controls water, metal controls wood, water controls fire.

This is also a fundamental balance because control means that one must keep in line, not oppress. A metal that excessively controls wood, which instead wants to expand, would suffocate its intrinsic nature and could therefore cause stagnation, a blockage of energy, an insecurity in expressing oneself... However, if this were to occur in an individual with a very strong wood- , at a certain point they would "explode" with all their yang, offending the grandfather, thus damaging the metal and causing further imbalances in the system: an excess of yang in the heart (schizophrenia) or an invasion of the earth (excessive control), preventing its function of transforming food, for example, and leading to gastric reflux.

In short, this law also highlights how the loss of overall balance can have consequences of various kinds and with different effects.

It is impossible to establish one effect for one cause. But this is not because we are talking about Chinese medicine, but because when we talk about a person's well-being, we are talking about biology, we are talking about complex systems where there are n factors that influence m organs and which can therefore generate n x m results, and all are interconnected and different effects can occur for each individual precisely because for each person an input can lead to different effects.

One center for everything

In all this, the earth has a rebalancing function, so the tendency should be to keep the earth strong and stable because it allows us to recover or mitigate the effects of a deficit in one of the movements. In the circular view, earth directly nourishes metal, but it is also the body's granary, and this makes it a privileged supplier of the kidney/water, which conserves and distributes yin/yang energies in the body, limits the expansion of wood, and mitigates the ardor of fire. So if you work on earth, you can't go wrong. In fact, reading inversely, if in doubt about what to work on, start with earth. But what does it mean to work on earth? It means 'centering': in the graphic representation of the cardinal points, fire is south, water is north, wood is east, metal is west, and earth is in the center. If an element is in excess or deficient, we will need to rectify the convergence of our being, our actions, and our emotions, and we will have to rebalance ourselves in the center.

It means "moderating" through flavors. Flavors are elements that influence the five movements and are used to correct excesses: bitter purifies fire, spicy energizes metal, salty nourishes the kidneys, sour contains wood, and sweet nourishes earth. Since flavors are used to correct excesses, we then need to stabilize ourselves at the center by adding a sweet flavor (which is not sugar but the flavor of boiled rice), which is suitable for all flavors.

It means 'to structure': fire controls the blood and blood vessels, and therefore the vitality of the individual; metal controls breathing and Qi; water controls fluids and bones; wood moves Qi in all directions and controls muscle tension through the tendons; earth builds the organs and muscles ( ). If energy is given by mass for acceleration (Qi), in our existence we must take care of both our Qi and our structure, but since transforming matter is a longer-term process than transforming energy, once again, earth becomes the element to which we must devote constant and continuous attention.

No prevalence

These are just a few examples of the reasoning behind the dynamics that link the various movements within our existence, whether we consider the more physical or the more intangible aspects. Once we enter into the perspective of reasoning about yin/yang balances and dynamics and the 5 movements, it will become much easier to learn about ourselves, others, and to live in harmony with the microcosm and macrocosm.

Above all, we must not fall into the typical Western error of becoming attached to a movement because it is "more beautiful, more interesting, the one that suits me." Another mistake is to think that you can perform all movements at 100% or even 110%. It is infinitely more important to have a balance between elements than to have a preponderance of one or two or to make an exhausting attempt to take these movements to extremes.

This will be better understood when we talk about Jing, but the issue is easily intuited: if an individual has a predominance of wood (say 90%) and 50% earth, 80% fire, and 40% metal, they will have to try to support the deficient elements and mitigate the effects of the dominant ones. This is because wood invades earth (and blocks it, preventing the transformation of liquids and food) and offends the grandfather (metal) by inhibiting the functions of this movement (respiratory function, depression, attachment). Therefore, it is much more important to bring all the elements to values of 70/75% and allow the individual to avoid imbalances. Because the elements, influencing each other in sustaining or consuming each other, will ultimately activate dynamics of consumption and absorption such that the final result will be to exhaust the weak elements and then draw on the strong elements and exhaust them prematurely as well.

Let us now review each of the 5 movements, giving a reading that is not too scientific but rather drawing on the ancient texts of the Huang di Nei Jing, also to learn to read through the metaphors with which the ancient masters taught their disciples through similes extrapolated from nature. and everyday life to recognize that the laws of the five movements are everywhere and relegating them to a few specific phenomena limits the individual's ability to recognize the universal laws that govern and organize the entire cosmos.

4.4 The Wood Movement

Wood Movement

In Heaven it is the wind,

on Earth it is wood,

in bodily structures it is the muscles,

in the zang it is the liver,

in the colored aspects it is blue-green,

in sounds it is the cry,

in movements reactive to an alteration it is the squeeze (contracture),

in the orifices it is the eye,

in flavors it is sour,

in desires it is anger.

Anger damages the Liver.

(Huangdi NeiJing Suwen, chapter 5)

Wood is an energy that rises and symbolizes rebirth, spring, and the force of nature. It is an energy that moves.

It is an upward growth movement, typical of trees. The branches of trees evoke the idea of flexibility (under the action of the wind). If our body and mind are flexible, we have good Wood energy.

It is connected to the muscles and tendons in their contractile function and in the generation of actual movement; on the other hand, the shape and trophism of the muscles is controlled by the spleen.

The Liver is in charge of commanding the army,

it analyzes the situation and plans strategies.

The gallbladder is responsible for what is right and correct,

issuing determination and decisions.

(Huangdi NeiJing Suwen, chap. 8)

Psyche and emotions

The Liver stores blood, and blood is the seat of the Hun.

When the Liver's breath is empty, there is fear;

when they are full, there is anger.

(Huangdi NeiJing Lingshu)

The psychic aspect of Wood influences our ability to make plans, take decisions (gallbladder), plan our lives, and give them meaning and direction. In fact, "The Liver is like an army general, who has a vision of strategy and the courage to go into battle to implement it." Furthermore, the free flow of Liver energy provides our mind with creativity and aspirations.

There are three Hun souls, which are related to the ability to remember images, to dream, and to plan. They reside in the Liver, where the abundance of blood provides them with a foundation and a stable home. They return to Heaven during sleep (and at the moment of death). It is during sleep, in fact, that these souls can roam freely and reach other souls: it is in this dream phase that we can reach high levels of perception and multidimensional and timeless communication.

The Hun are our Ethereal Soul (as opposed to the Po, which are our bodily souls).

If the Liver is weak, its psychic aspect (Hun) is not rooted: it begins to wander through space and time, generating fear and a lack of direction in life. It is not rooted and hallucinations of any kind may occur, as well as a desire to fly: the hun would try to manifest itself even when awake.

Wood does not like compression (its energy is to rise and expand); if it is exercised, it can become unbalanced. This manifests itself through anger, resentment, and frustration: emotions that will hurt the Liver. To manage them, we can help ourselves with breathing exercises!

Food and nutrition

Problematic foods for this movement are:

- too much animal-based and salty food,

- too many baked goods,

- too much fat

- too much sugar (sucrose, but also fructose, which could cause steatosis, or fatty liver).

Coffee (roasting could burden the energy of the Liver/Gallbladder) and alcohol (it's still sugar!) can also contribute to worsening the condition of Wood.

The recommendation is to eat green foods (green leafy vegetables): green is the color of the Liver.

A moderately sour taste (such as lemon or umeboshi) can help us. On the other hand, an excess of acid in intensity (foods that are too acidic, such as vinegar) and quantity could harm the liver as they are astringent and would therefore compress and limit the expansive energy of wood.

A balanced sweet flavor (such as that of well-chewed whole grains) also tones the energy of the liver.

Temperament

According to Sun Si Miao, temperament is the energy level most closely connected to Yuan Qi, which is the original energy, and is therefore linked to our constitution. The other levels are emotions and feelings (Ying level) and sensations (Wei level). By knowing our temperament, we know ourselves. Sometimes external conditions influence the individual, favoring the manifestation of characteristics that do not originally belong to them, i.e., they are acquired. It is through the study of the original temperament that a person's true temperament can be identified.

Wood represents the relationship with the outside world, openness, extroversion, assertiveness, and the ability to express oneself. Shy and introverted people are deficient in the expression of wood.

Movement and physical activity

Movement and physical activity aim to focus attention on what is appropriate based on the individual's temperament or the season. It is good to follow one's own nature (temperament), but it is also good to experience other natures in order to balance all energy movements, be ready, and understand when to devote oneself to an energy lodge because it needs to be supported and when not to. Furthermore, according to Chinese medicine, physical activities should be practiced to maintain good health, strengthen the weakest parts, and never exhaust energy or stress all or part of the body, even from an emotional point of view. For this reason, competitive activity is not covered in this discussion. This does not mean that it is forbidden, but since the level of stress that professional athletes are subjected to is very high, progressive, continuous, and comprehensiv l preparation is necessary, involving every physical and energetic level. This means strengthening muscles, tendons, and bones, but also balance, coordination, proprioception, anxiety management, breathing, listening to one's blood flow, and managing anger, disappointment, sadness, friendship, sharing, and respect. Needless to say, what matters today is performance, in a short time and without too much respect for the opponent, but these are the times we live in; however, you can always choose to practice without the goal of winning.

The movement of wood is expansion, but wood generally requires movement. So even just walking helps wood, preferably in nature where the presence of green helps and nourishes the energy of this movement. However, the ideal would be to do at least medium-intensity physical activity that involves accelerated breathing: prolonged or endurance work may be recommended; it also helps us to understand our abilities and energy levels, so that once I have a goal, I will have the vision and create the appropriate strategy to achieve it. In this way, we also act on the diaphragm, an organ connected to the liver and blood, where emotions are blocked: when wood allows Qi to flow freely, emotions are no longer trapped. Wood wants to expand in all directions, so it is good to do activities and exercises that involve the lower and upper limbs as well as the trunk (the name itself should suggest something), in the open air and involving sweating, to eliminate accumulated toxins. Martial arts are the activities that best express the wood element.

Element	WOOD
Organ	Liver
Viscera	Gallbladder
Season	Spring
Quadrant	East
Planet	Jupiter
Action of the season	Generate
Color	Green - blue
Numbers	3 and 8
Reactive movement	Squeeze
Atmospheric breath	Wind (feng)
Body parts	Tendons - movement
Orifice	Eyes
Own spirit	Souls (Hun)
Emotions or expressions of will	Impetuosity - anger
Taste	Acid
Organic fluid	Tears
Sound emitted from the throat	Scream
Musical note	3rd note
Virtue	Humanity (ren)
Smell	Rancid
Cereal	Wheat
Domestic animal	Chicken
Outward display of splendor	Nails

4.5 Fire movement

Fire movement

In Heaven it is heat,

on Earth there is fire,

in bodily structures it is the mai (vessels),

in the zang it is the heart,

in the colored aspects it is red,

in sounds it is laughter,

in movement reactive to an alteration it is dejection,

in the orifices it is the tongue,

in flavors it is bitterness,

in desires it is joy.

Joy (when exaggerated: agitation) damages the heart.

(Huangdi NeiJing Suwen, chap. 5)

Fire represents the moment of maximum expansion. Its nature is to rise, produce heat, and illuminate. It is the root of life and the origin of mental life.

The Heart has the power of lord and master,

it emanates the splendor of the Spirits (Shen).

The small intestine is responsible for receiving and prospering, releases the transformed substances.

(Huangdi NeiJing Suwen, chap. 8)

The Heart is the sovereign, the king. Its mode of government is determined by non-action (wu-wei), which does not mean doing nothing: it is, in fact, the ability to allow each being to develop according to the gifts and talents inherent in each.

The Small Intestine is the organ (viscera) that separates the Pure from the Impure and makes choices. It is responsible for protecting the self. This task is not limited to the body, but also extends to the mind: the intestine influences our ability to make decisions (even if it is the Gallbladder that ultimately decides), to see clearly, providing us with the elements to evaluate situations in life before making our decisions (Gallbladder) and acting (Liver).

If the intestine is out of balance, we lose our mental clarity and our ability to evaluate, both physically and psychologically. In this case, the intestine loses its ability to choose, letting everything pass. For example, leaky gut syndrome is quite common today.

Psyche and emotions

The heart treasures the network of animation that is the seat of the spirits (Shen).

When the heart's breaths are empty, there is sadness;

when they are full, we laugh without being able to stop.

52

(Huangdi NeiJing Lingshu)

According to Traditional Chinese Medicine, mental activities and consciousness reside in the Heart, which influences our emotions and houses the Shen, responsible for affectivity, thought, consciousness, memory (of distant events), and sleep.

The Shen corresponds to the Mind and is related to the Heart, but it also includes all the other emotions (mental and spiritual) of the other organs, namely

Hun (Ethereal Soul), which resides in the Liver

Yi (Intellect), which resides in the Spleen

Po (Corporeal Soul), which resides in the Lungs

Zhi (Will), which resides in the Kidneys

The heart carries our emotions and provides us with insight, the ability to perceive. Let's think about the etymology of the word Intelligence: it comes from the Latin intus-legere, which means to read inside. We can say that intelligence is the faculty that allows us to know. It is from the Heart that our ability to relate, communicate, listen empathically, and perceive derives.

For this reason, the Heart is defined as the Emperor of the Internal Organs and is also called "the root of Life."

The state of the Heart and Blood will influence our emotions and our mind. If the heart is weak and the blood is deficient (unable to anchor the Shen), we may experience mental problems, depression, poor memory, insomnia or drowsiness, a scattered mind, and even loss of consciousness.

The heart controls speech. Stuttering, as well as the tendency to talk a lot, can be related to an imbalance of the heart.

Joy is the emotion connected to the Heart. An excess of emotions can fatigue the Heart. The Shen, in fact, love calm and quiet; if human beings are "in a state of cheerfulness and joy, they become frightened and disperse, leaving the heart."

Food

From a nutritional point of view, a balanced diet is always the most recommended.

On the other hand, a diet with too much fat, salt (especially if of poor quality), refined products, and alcohol will damage the condition of the Heart. This corresponds, in fact, to the picture of modern nutrition. It is no coincidence that cardiovascular diseases are currently one of the main problems in healthcare.

The flavor of the heart is bitter. A balanced bitterness (bitter vegetables) nourishes it. An excess of this flavor will contribute to creating imbalance.

Similarly, foods such as sugar, tropical foods, and an excess of spices will disperse our mind.

Temperament

The temperament of the fire individual is the measure of the intensity of their emotions. It is the tendency to dramatize, to be very anxious, emotional, reactive, or neurotic. It is also the characteristic of being pleasant and sensual.

Movement and physical activity

The movement of fire is elevation, but in general, fire is movement, dance, striving upwards. There is explosiveness, there is a peak of energy to be expressed but without completely exhausting it: fire must be tamed without suffocating it. The art of fire is the secret of alchemy and leads to the greatest results if the right compromise can be found. Therefore, fire requires an almost competitive activity, but not one aimed at exhausting energy. In any case, it is the exaltation of Shen, which encompasses all knowledge of technique, perception of one's body, grace, and beauty. If you go running, there is a training program behind it to improve your performance, or to strengthen your cardiovascular system, and so on. The ideal would be to do high-intensity physical activity—but not endurance—or artistic activity. So movement, but also creativity, such as tennis, artistic gymnastics, or skating. At the end of the activity, there should be no feeling of exhaustion, disorientation, or confusion, but rather joy, happiness, and a sense of progress. It is important not to seriously affect (even if only temporarily) the yin (blood, fluids, marrow), so it is important to stay hydrated and not push yourself to

Element	FIRE
Organ	Heart - Pericardium
Viscera	Small intestine - Triple heater
Season	Summer
Quadrant	South
Planet	Mars
Seasonal action	Grow
Color	Red
Numbers	2 and 7
Reactive movement	Oppression
Atmospheric pressure	Heat
Parts of the body	Energy and vital channels
Orifice	Tongue
Own spirit	Shen
Emotions or expressions of will	Happiness and joy
Taste	Bitter (ku)
Organic fluid	Sweat
Sound emitted from the throat	Laughter
Musical note	4th note
Virtue	Sense of rituals
Smell	Burnt
Cereal	Glutinous millet
Domestic animal	Ram
Outward manifestation of splendor	Complexion and face

exhaustion.

4.6 Earth movement

Earth movement

In Heaven it is moisture,

on Earth it is earth,

in bodily structures it is flesh

in the zang it is the spleen,

in the colored aspects it is yellow,

in sounds it is singing,

in movements reactive to an alteration it is belching,

in the orifices it is the mouth,

in flavors it is sweetness,

in desires it is thought.

Thought causes damage to the spleen.

(Huangdi NeiJing Suwen, chap. 5)

The characteristic of this movement is to welcome, generate, and nourish.

It is the place where everything is welcomed, processed, digested, transformed. It is the energy of support, of rooting. It produces all forms. It dispenses life. It nourishes us, like a mother.

In the cycle of the five movements, Earth is at the center: it distributes the energy that allows the movements to relate and transform. Even in the seasons, it is represented as the period of transition (eighteen days) between one season and another. It is also associated with the late summer period.

The Spleen and Stomach are in charge of barns and granaries, emanating the Five Flavors.

(Huangdi NeiJing Suwen, chap. 8)

The Stomach receives food and digests it. The Spleen transforms it and makes it assimilable by the body. It extracts the Jing—the essence—of food and distributes it to all the organs.

The spleen directs gu Qi (the pure energy of food) upwards to the lungs, where it combines with air to form chest energy (zong Qi, which descends to the kidneys and strengthens our vital energy) and to the heart to form blood. It provides us with nourishing energy: what in Traditional Chinese Medicine is called the energy of the Posterior Heaven (which, together with the energy of the Anterior Heaven that we receive at birth, is stored in the Kidneys).

Psyche and emotions

The spleen treasures reconstruction, which is the seat of purpose.

58

(Huangdi NeiJing Lingshu)

Purpose (Yi) is our ability to digest and assimilate, not only physically but also psychologically: to analyze, process, evaluate, and reorganize concepts and ideas. It is the ability to become aware of oneself and turn this awareness into purpose and intention.

The spleen is home to the intellect, responsible for concentration, memory, focusing our thoughts, and our reflection.

From an emotional point of view, it is empathy, the ability to relate to others, to detach ourselves from our ego in order to welcome, sympathize, feel with others, share the feelings of others, and give without reserve.

The spleen controls the five flavors (sweet, bitter, sour, spicy, salty), extracting them from food and distributing them to the five organs. Each organ-movement is associated with a flavor, in such a way as to allow balance (according to the principle of Traditional Chinese Medicine). Therefore, the Liver-Wood, which is a movement of expansion, is associated with the sour taste, which has a restraining action. Sweet is associated with the Spleen-Earth, bitter with the Heart-Fire, spicy with the Lung-Metal, and salty with the Kidney-Water. In Traditional Chinese Medicine, flavor is a form of energy and nourishment: it nourishes the organ, provided it is consumed in moderate quantities and intensity. Thus, sweetness nourishes the spleen, provided it is balanced, such as the sweetness of cooked and well-chewed cereal. Otherwise, an intense, un r flavor such as that of sugar (or worse, fructose) will harm this organ.

An energy imbalance in this movement can manifest itself in a thought that remains stuck; thinking of a loop can give an idea of this: a repetitive thought that moves in circles without finding a way out.

These obsessive thoughts generate worry and can, in turn, damage the spleen.

They are often accompanied by eating disorders (anorexia, bulimia, orthorexia).

Food

Today's diet certainly offers us more opportunities for imbalance. In addition to the quantity of food (which is considerable nowadays), the food we consume today is extremely poor in quality: it is often industrially processed (and therefore refined), out of season, not local, and grown with synthetic products. This causes foods to lose all their Jing energy.

The spleen hates moisture, which interferes with its transformation and distribution activities. An excess of raw and cold foods (raw vegetables and cheese) can create moisture accumulation.

We have also seen that an excessively sweet taste (such as that of sugar) can alter the functions of the spleen. Our emotional stability, in fact, depends on the stability of blood sugar, whose fluctuations make us feel very excited (hyperglycemia) or very depressed (hypoglycemia).

Even a taste that is too sour can create imbalances in the spleen.

Highly contractive foods (such as excess salt and animal products, but also an abuse of 'dry' cooking styles) can dry out the 'Earth' too much, producing hard 'dry clods' and creating transformation: even our thinking can become rigid and stagnant, generating an imbalance in the spleen.

Our diet should be varied, with fresh, unprocessed food, balanced between Yin and Yang, balanced in cooking styles and with respect to the five flavors (bitter, sweet, spicy, salty, sour), so as to harmoniously nourish all the organs.

Temperament

The earth individual is linked to the ability to be accommodating, to put people at ease. This is a typical characteristic of the healer, because it is necessary for the therapist (earth) to get along and be in tune/empathy/harmony with those who turn to them.

Movement and physical activity

The movement of earth tends towards stabilization, so the physical activity that nourishes this element is strengthening, stabilizing, and increasing in intensity to reinforce the muscular and tendon structure: the aim is to increase mass but in a balanced way, as it should be, without hypertrophy. No part of the body is favored over others, but the focus of movement and stability lies in the center, the trunk. Any exercise that improves balance, strengthens and increases muscle mass, perfects posture, and develops coordination without disrupting the metabolism is recommended. The body should not be pushed to exhaustion and must always be hydrated. Endurance activities are not suitable for wood, but rather all forms of gymnastics, dance, taiji, and yoga. The whole body occupies the space, there is no preference for high or low, but the center, and in the center the individual is a rock. The development of the motor skills of the earth allows for specialization in specific disciplines. At the end of the activity, you feel strong, stable, and serene.

Element	EARTH
Organ	Spleen/Pancreas
Viscera	Stomach

Season	Intermediate season
Quadrant	Center
Planet	Saturn
Action of the season	Transform
Color	Yellow
Numbers	5 and 10
Reactive movement	Erupt
Atmospheric blow	Humidity
Body parts	Meat
Orifice	Mouth
Own spirit	Purpose - intention (yi)
Emotions or expressions of will	Obsessive thought (si)
Taste	Sweet (gan)
Organic fluid	Saliva
Sound emitted from the throat	Singing
Musical note	1st note
Virtue	Reliability
Smell	Flavored - fragrant - floral - fruity
Cereal	Non-glutinous millet
Domestic animal	Ox
Manifestation of splendor toward the outside world	Lips

4.7 Metal movement

Metal Movement

In Heaven it is dry,

on Earth it is metal,

in bodily structures it is the skin and hair,

in the zang organs it is the lungs,

in colored aspects it is white,

in sounds it is hiccups,

in movements reactive to an alteration it is coughing,

in the orifices it is the nose,

in flavors it is acrid,

in desires it is despondency.

Dejection damages the lungs.

(Huangdi NeiJing Suwen, chap. 5)

This is the energy of Heaven entering the Earth and condensing.

Metal is cold and hard: in humans, these qualities are expressed in the ability to detach oneself from things. Metal is shiny: our ability to bring clarity.

It is the energy of exchange: it allows us to relate to the outside world. It is our ability to accept and let go. To accept what comes to us from outside. To let go of what we do not need.

It corresponds to the West, to autumn, to the moment when we gather the fruits of the day (or year) and prepare for the rest of the night (or winter), so that we can wake up the next morning (or in spring).

The Lung has the role of minister and chancellor.

The Large Intestine is responsible for transit, expelling the residues of transformations.

(Huangdi NeiJing Suwen, chap. 8)

From a physiological point of view, the task of the Lungs is to bring in oxygen (for the blood to transport it throughout the body) and expel carbon dioxide.

Through breathing, the lungs connect us to the outside world. Breathing is the first act we perform at birth: by inhaling, we enter into communication with the new world.

By exhaling, we let go of matter to enter a new dimension. At death, our Corporeal Soul (Po) remains attached to the bones and returns to the Earth; our Ethereal Soul (Hun) ascends to Heaven.

Like the lungs, the large intestine is connected to exchange and is related to elimination. It is no coincidence that when we are unable to let go of emotions, for example, our intestines tend to somatize.

Another organ connected to exchange is the Skin: this is the largest organ we have and the one that eliminates the most. Through the skin (sweat) we also expel what is good to let go of, such as toxins.

Psyche and emotions

The lungs store the breath, which is the seat of the Po.

(Huangdi NeiJing Lingshu)

In psychological terms, breathing allows us to metabolize the outside world and bring it inside us, putting us in touch with our internal environment (introspection), acquiring perception of ourselves, and offering us the opportunity to get to know ourselves.

This energetic movement allows us to internalize meaningful experiences and let go of the superfluous. Only in this way (by eliminating and letting go) can we make room for new experiences and knowledge, and continue on our evolutionary path.

If the lungs and large intestine are out of balance, there is a risk of losing the exchange function and becoming stuck, closed in on ourselves, generating despondency, sadness, and melancholy. This attitude of closure can also manifest itself through our posture (closed shoulders, hunched forward).

Food

66

To keep the lungs healthy, it is best to avoid excessive dryness (which dries out the mucus, whose function is to protect the mucous membranes) and humidity (which could clog the lungs and congest the large intestine). It is advisable not to eat too many dry foods (dry and hard foods), avoiding a diet rich in refined and fatty foods, especially saturated fats.

Foods with contracting energy, such as excess salt and animal products, could create a closing movement for this organ.

The associated flavor is pungent, or spicy, which can counteract the closing of metal. It is a flavor that can penetrate and let go. Think, for example, of the flavor of ginger.

One particular precaution (which our body requires us to take in order to maintain balance) is to adapt our diet to the climate and the seasons. During the summer, to cope with the intense heat, we tend to eat more refreshing foods. In autumn (the season of Metal), we should try to let go of the cold (our body no longer needs it) to make room for more warming foods, recreating the internal-external balance (cold outside, warm inside). If this does not happen, if we are unable to eliminate what is no longer useful, our body will do it for us: illnesses such as colds serve this purpose (to expel the cold inside us through the elimination of mucus).

Brown rice is one of the best foods for the lungs and large intestine.

Temperament

Individuals with a metal temperament are organized, with the ability to set the right priorities and always do the right or best thing. They are hard workers, respectable and extremely reliable people.

Movement and physical activity

Metal is the introduction of yin, so there is a tendency to reduce the emphasis on expansion in favor of focusing on oneself. Activities that lead to reflection, silence, and contemplation, even lasting many hours. In autumn, we eliminate unnecessary things and look within ourselves, we look close to ourselves and, coincidentally, in autumn we can go on excursions in the woods and look for mushrooms, close to our feet or nearby, we can take long walks in the snow when it appears, enveloped in the muffled silence it gives us (, white is the color of metal), so activities in the snow such as walking, ski mountaineering, or snowshoeing nourish metal, both for their colors and for the introspective nature of the activity, the contemplation. It is good to do outdoor activities to prepare the lungs for the cold, but without letting yourself be attacked by cold winds, or indoors, but since the lungs love dryness, it is good for the air to be recycled.

Element	METAL
Organ	Lungs
Viscera	Large intestine
Season	Autumn
Quadrant	West
Planet	Venus
Seasonal action	Harvest
Color	White
Numbers	4 and 9
Reactive movement	Cough
Atmospheric breath	Dryness
Body parts	Skin and hair
Orifice	Nose
Spirit	Souls (Po)
Emotions or expressions of will	Reflection and sadness
Taste	Spicy
Organic fluid	Nasal mucus
Sound emitted from the throat	Hiccups
Musical note	2nd note
Virtue	Sense of duty and justice
Smell	Rotten
Cereal	Rice
Pet	Horse
Outward manifestation	Hair

4.8 Water movement

Water movement

In Heaven it is cold,

on Earth it is water,

in bodily structures it is bones,

in the zang organs it is the kidneys,

in the colored aspects it is black,

in sounds it is the sigh,

in movement reactive to an alteration it is the shiver,

in the orifices it is the ear,

in flavors it is saltiness,

in desires it is fear.

Fear damages the kidneys.

(Huangdi NeiJing Suwen, chap. 5)

Water is a very profound energy: it constitutes the beginning and end of every process in human beings. It is the energy that is provided to us at the moment of conception. It is infinite potentiality.

The kidneys are responsible for arousing power,

they emanate skill and savoir-faire.

The bladder is responsible for territories and cities,

and stores bodily fluids.

(Huangdi NeiJing Suwen, chap. 8)

This is where we accumulate our vital force. The kidneys store Jing, the essence of the Front Heaven (i.e., what we inherit, which determines our basic constitution) and the Back Heaven (the essence extracted from food and air).

The Jing of the Front Heaven is like a battery that is given to us at birth. Our lifespan and good health depend on its characteristics. Based on our lifestyle and dietary choices, we can determine, over the years, whether it is consumed slowly or quickly.

We can choose to dissipate as little of this energy as possible, drawing on the energy of the chest (through proper breathing) and food (energy processed by the stomach and spleen).

In the macrocosm, the corresponding season is winter: in nature, everything is internalized, everything is reduced to the essential. Plants shed their leaves and appear dead, but in reality, sap has accumulated inside to collect energy and release it later.

In space, it is the North: it is associated with the North Star.

The kidneys generate marrow, which in turn nourishes the bones, giving them strength and elasticity. If there is a kidney deficiency, marrow is scarce and the bones will no longer be properly nourished and . Spontaneous fractures (e.g., in the elderly) can be attributed to a deficiency of Kidney Jing. If we want strong bones and to prevent (especially for women) osteoporosis problems, we should try not to damage our Kidneys and provide them with the right nutrition.

Teeth, hair, and reproductive organs are also connected to the kidneys.

Psyche and emotions

The kidneys store essences, which are the seat of Will.

(Huangdi NeiJing Lingshu)

Associated with the kidneys is Will (Zhi). If our kidneys are strong, our willpower will be strong. I want, therefore I am. Here we find our self, the deepest part of us. In its deep waters we find the unconscious. It is the energy that provides us with existential drive, willpower, and determination. It gives us structure and strength, supporting us in times of stress. If we are in balance, our self will be well structured and we will be confident. Otherwise, we will be pervaded by insecurity and fears, even if they are unfounded.

Water also provides us with wisdom, the ability to adapt, to flow.

Apathy, listlessness, and panic attacks can be traced back to an imbalance of Water.

Food

The kidneys are healthy if water can flow. Excessive cold can freeze water, creating stagnation.

What can harm this organ are foods that are too cold, too sweet (sugar, fructose, etc.), and an excess of protein.

It is important not to eat too much (overeating damages the kidneys) or too little (otherwise, we may be forced to draw on our inherited Jing reserves, reducing them).

The kidneys are nourished by the energy linked to the lungs. If we eat foods that clog the lungs, we will not be able to properly nourish the energy of the kidneys. We should therefore pay particular attention to refined and fatty foods (especially saturated fats), which can create excess mucus, clog the lungs, and prevent the kidneys from being properly nourished.

Winter is the season when we need to take special care of our kidneys, which are sensitive to the cold. During this period, we should try to avoid cold and cooling foods, preferring double cooking or long cooking times such as stews (nishime).

We nourish our kidneys through seeds: whole grains, legumes—especially beans (which, not coincidentally, resemble small kidneys). We can also help ourselves with roots, condiments, and fermented s such as miso or tamari, good quality salt (whole sea salt, to be used sparingly), and seaweed (especially kombu).

Temperament

The temperament of the water individual is defined as 'kai fang', which means 'openness' (kai) and 'letting things be as they are' (fang), i.e. the ability to adapt to situations, just as water takes the shape of the container into which it is poured, whether it is a round, square or elliptical jug.

Movement and physical activity

Finally, water, winter. You need to treasure your energy, stop the phase of reflection, and calm the waves of thoughts. Meditation, some types of yoga that are not too extreme, Qigong, and here too, walking and skiing. Anything that strengthens the legs and lower back is recommended, as is swimming, which takes place in the water element. But don't overdo it; sweating too much is not recommended. You need to move your Qi, but gently, making small waves without creating foam. Energy must be preserved both because the next season—spring—needs resources to explode with all its emphasis, and because the seasons of life – both the pre- and neonatal phases and old age – see us limited in our motor skills and unable to waste fundamental energies, and also be , because individuals with a water temperament will not have overly dynamic characteristics and attitudes and must not upset them, as this would deeply damage their essence, the balance of their energies, and their bones.

Element	WATER
Organ	Kidneys
Viscera	Bladder
Season	Winter
Quadrant	North
Planet	Mercury

Action of the season	Hoard
Color	Black
Numbers	1 and 6
Reactive movement	Shiver
Atmospheric breath	Cold
Body parts	Bones and marrow
Orifice	Ears or lower orifices
Own spirit	Wanting (zhi)
Emotions or expressions of will	Meditation and Fear (kong)
Taste	Salty (xian)
Organic fluid	Spit
Sound emitted from the throat	Sighs
Musical note	5th note
Virtue	Wisdom (zhi)
Smell	Fermented, putrid
Cereal	Bean
Domestic animal	Pig
Manifestation of outward splendor	Hair and teeth

Below is a brief summary of the relationships between the various movements and their positioning within space and the seasons, useful for understanding when one is most stressed and at what stage one can work to strengthen one rather than the other.

ELEMENT	WOOD	FIRE	EARTH	METAL
ORGAN	Liver (gan)	Heart (xin)	Spleen (pi)	Lung (fei)
DIRECTION	East	South	Center	West
SEASON	Spring	Summer	Intermediate seasons	Fall
MOTHER	Water	Wood	Fire	Earth

(nourished by)				
SON (nourishes)	Fire	Earth	Metal	Water
CONTROL	Earth	Metal	Water	Wood
CONTROLLED BY	Metal	Aqua	Wood	Fire

5. SAN BAO: JING, QI, AND SHEN

5.1 Definition and meaning of San Bao

I believe that certain Chinese terms are necessary to better understand some principles of Chinese medicine. One of these is "San Bao," or the three treasures, which refer to Jing, Qi, and Shen. These are the most important energetic elements of our existence, and one could discuss them at length for thousands of pages, but I will try to summarize the principles and functions of these elements.

To address the topic of San Bao, however, we must also introduce the concept of Dan Tien, which is the chamber of alchemical transformation. What does this mean? It means that our body has three areas dedicated to the accumulation and transformation of San Bao energies. We therefore have the lower Dan Tien, located in the abdomen, approximately below the navel, the middle Dan Tien, located in the rib cage in the area of the heart and lungs, and finally the upper Dan Tien located in the skull. Each Dan Tien stores and transforms one of the San Bao: the lower Dan Tien has Jing, the middle Dan Tien has Qi, and the upper Dan Tien has Shen.

5.2 Jing: The Vital Essence

Jing represents the densest form of energy available to us and has a dual nature: prenatal and postnatal. The prenatal form is defined as the anterior heaven and consists of the genetic, energetic, and karmic makeup provided by the parents at the moment of conception.

The stronger and healthier the parents are at the moment of conception, the stronger the Jing of the child will be. It is therefore the biological inheritance that is passed on from parents to children. This form of Jing cannot be regenerated, so if it is completely consumed, the person will be in a state of substantial weakness.

Then there is postnatal Jing, from the posterior sky, which is the nourishment available to the individual during their lifetime and which can partially regenerate and nourish them thanks to 'nutrients': air, food, rest, and positive emotions. Postnatal Jing is drawn on before prenatal Jing, so before the 'roots' are affected, this type of Jing must be consumed, meaning that unless the individual decides to lead an extremely wasteful lifestyle, they will always be able to limit the damage. It should be noted that Jing is depleted when one leads a very wasteful lifestyle: this includes an unrestrained sex life, very tiring and/or very stressful work, and insufficient nutrition (as defined above) for the h , which depletes reserves. We must think of Jing as the oil in a lamp that must be used sparingly so that it lasts as long as possible without wasting resources.

Jing consists of two parts: the first means food, cereals (and generally refers to rice), the second means 'will to live'. Jing is therefore the dense part that is formed and maintained by food and which preserves within itself the desire for incarnation in human beings, a desire that can be transferred by producing offspring. A healthy and strong Jing can be identified by appetite and the desire to live and/or procreate. This is one of the few alchemical interpretations that can be found in Chinese medicine books.

5.3 Qi: Vital Energy

Qi is perhaps the best-known term, but it is also the most debated. Without getting into very complex philosophical or scientific arguments, we can say that Qi is the energy that enlivens and animates an individual. There are also different types of Qi based on density and function: Yuan Qi (which derives directly from Jing and nourishes the organs), Yin Qi (which comes from food), Yang Qi (which is voluntary and involuntary motor energy), and Wei Qi (the defensive energy of the immune system, which is the least dense). Let's say that if the ultimate goal is the psychophysical well-being of the person, it is necessary to have a good level of Wei Qi, which represents the strength of the immune system but is also the energy that flows in the tendino-muscular meridians, so when Wei Qi is abundant, our immune system works well but also our musculoskeletal system is in good condition.

Qi is the real energy and is nourished by the transformation of the foods mentioned above. When accumulated, they increase postnatal Jing.

The energy we need to live and carry out our individual activities is therefore Qi. If we do not eat enough, we become deficient in Qi and deplete our reserves of postnatal Jing. Continuing with this pattern of excessive consumption will also deplete postnatal Jing and draw on prenatal Jing reserves. The evidence of this energy depletion in some individuals is easily identifiable: signs of fatigue, posture, dullness in the eyes, graying hair, weak teeth and bones... It is not easy to understand which type of Jing is being depleted, but our body gives us indications if we are "overdoing" or "doing something wrong" in our lifestyle. If the signs of decay/fatigue disappear within a few days, thanks to rest, proper nutrition, and appropriate physical activity, it means that we were consuming all our Qi. If, on the other hand, a few days are not enough and there are significant signs (which can also be detected through blood tests, for example), it means that Jing has been affected. Autoimmune diseases, which have become the norm in our society , are certainly difficult to reverse, which means that they have affected the deep structure, if not the DNA itself: these are signs of Jing depletion.

In the example of the oil lamp, Qi is comparable to the heat and movement of the flame. If I exaggerate the power, I will get a very strong flame, but I will then consume the oil prematurely.

5.4 Shen: the Spirit

Shen is normally translated as 'spirit' and is also divided into two types: Great Shen and Small Shen. Great Shen is the principle that governs the universe, the Word in our Christian tradition. It is the input of all that exists and is the input that rains down on the embryo when parents conceive their children: it is the element that meets Jing and enlivens it and gives it a mandate, a destiny. The individual forgets this once the body comes to life, but it is something they should realize in this existence in order to return and reunite with the Great Shen.

We can therefore attribute the most spiritual aspect to this energetic element. Shen dwells in the heart but expresses itself through the upper Dan Tian (the skull). In fact, the sense organs (which have openings to the outside world in the skull) are called "the orifices of the heart" and represent the sensory instruments through which we receive stimuli from external reality that are "translated" and reported to Shen (which dwells in the heart). Shen therefore refers to the more ethereal, more yang part, if we want to define it according t l dualistic principles of Taoism, but like every aspect of Chinese medicine, it is not limited to having only spiritual or psychological effects. Of course, a restless soul, a restless Shen, can be seen in behavior, in attitude, in something that is not tangible. However, in the long run, it also influences the material part. A 'dull' Shen leads to a lack of energy, depression, and certainly posture will suffer the consequences. The same is true of an excited Shen (perhaps caused by drug use): you see? A material substance ingested has effects on the immaterial Shen, which over time leads to effects on Qi (energy depletion) and Jing (organ depletion).

The Shen, in the example of the lamp, is the light: the ultimate purpose for which we use the oil lamp, because if we needed to warm ourselves, we would have lit the fireplace. Instead, we want to light our way... back home... and we need a light that does not burn out quickly because the journey is not a short one. And the heat of the flame (Qi) is not superfluous, because through Qi and its good use we can have different experiences in this existence (the heat that warms us, the heat that warms the food we eat, the heat that evaporates water or melts ice): heat is the manifestation of life in this body and in this world.

5.5 Xue and Jin ye

In Chinese medicine, blood is called Xue and, compared to our concept of blood, it takes on a broader meaning. The adage says: "Qi moves and warms, Xue nourishes and moisturizes." This is to remember the basic functions of these two elements, which are key to the health of our body. The yang aspect (Qi) and the yin aspect (Xue). In fact, Xue is the fluid pumped by the heart to all organs and body parts to nourish and hydrate every single cell. When there is a deficiency of yin, there is probably a deficiency of

Xue. When there is an excess of yang, it consumes yin and therefore also Xue, which may be too little or too dense. In any case, it has no strength, no nourishment, does not moisturize, and does not nourish the organs, thus compromising the yin of our body. Qi is closely linked to Xue in that its energy pushes it into the body, thanks to the thrust provided by the lungs: Qi is said to be the rider of Xue. Lungs, Qi, and Xue: this helps us understand why long, deep breathing allows the lungs to fill up and have enough Qi to push blood throughout the body without accelerating the heartbeat: it increases the intensity but not the frequency.

Jin ye, on the other hand, are all the other organic fluids in our body: juices, secretions, joint fluids, urine, connective tissue fluids, and semen. They too have a varied h I function in the body, nourishing, lubricating, conveying the expulsion of Qi and toxic substances, and have different densities. There are five Jin ye that require attention, also from an energy diagnosis perspective, and they are associated with the five organs: sweat – heart; mucus or nasal secretions – lungs; tears – liver; saliva – spleen; thick saliva – kidneys. Fluids must flow, and when they thicken, they can cause stagnation, blockages, and interference in the circulation of Qi. One of the most harmful fluids is tan (phlegm), which is catarrh (but not only nasal). In fact, at the lung level, it causes coughing, mucus, and dyspnea. in the meridians, tan causes blockages, hemiplegia, paralysis, and pain; in the heart, it causes palpitations, agitation, and mental disorders; in the head and marrow, it causes dizziness, vertigo, headache, and heaviness.

A good balance requires sufficient yin (fluids and blood to nourish and moisturize) without exaggeration, because too much yin cools the yang and therefore there would be a deficiency of Qi (which warms the organs and moves fluids), which can lead to edema and, in the long run, tan. However, an excess of yang also leads to an excess of Qi and heat, which consumes the liquid part of substances, leaving the denser part, and therefore tan can form without there being edema.

Finally, let us not forget that Xue is closely linked to Shen: in fact, Shen is rooted in Xue. If Xue is scarce or lacking in vitality, Shen risks having no roots and ting to detach itself to reach the great Shen. It may not succeed, but serious mental disorders can occur, and this shows us how Chinese medicine managed to understand, thousands of years ago, the correlation between mental problems arising from physical causes—a correlation that our modern, pharmacological medicine has not yet managed to grasp.

5.6 Full and empty

We intend to conclude the theoretical part of this compendium with a very important concept that has been deliberately left to the end to allow for a better understanding of this concept, which is both energetic and material, but also philosophical and spiritual. Therefore, everyone can expand their reading of the concept of 'full and empty' on all levels of their existence.

Full refers to a state of saturation that tends towards excess. Whether it is Yang or Yin (when one of the two energies exceeds the threshold of personal balance (sunstroke, cold, consumption of ice-cold drinks, etc.). But fullness can also affect the energy of individual movements: excess Yang in the liver (Yang of wood) leading to angry reactions (emotional level) or gastric reflux (physical level)... Although excess may seem positive in our capitalist, resource-accumulating culture, it can cause a blockage of functionality and impede the flow of activities d in the correct order. Let's imagine accumulating goods and storing them in the entrance to our home. After a while, there will be so much stuff that it will be difficult to move around easily and go to other rooms. An excess must therefore be 'drained' to restore the right energy level.

Emptiness, as you will intuitively understand, represents a deficiency, Yin, Yang or, as mentioned above, a lack of energy in one of the elements, for example, a deficiency of lung Qi (shortness of breath, asthma, weak voice, asthenia). Undoubtedly, a deficiency is easier to identify and treat because it may be more obvious if something is missing and therefore what is needed to increase it. However, it is always necessary to trace back to what caused that deficiency because if it is caused by an excess of another energy, until the excess is drained and the balance is restored, any addition of what is deficient will only bring temporary benefits.

We would also like to offer a spiritual insight into the importance of emptiness: a Zen story tells of a traveler who went to a famous master to achieve enlightenment. The master agreed to meet him and they sat down at a table set for tea tasting. They began to talk, then the master took the teapot and poured tea into the traveler's cup, which was already full. He was astonished and irritated because the spilled tea had wet him. He got up and left. Shortly afterwards, however, he thought about the scene and returned and found the master still sitting at the table. He took the cup, emptied it, and said, "Excuse me, master, now my cup is empty, I can receive your tea." The empty cup is our mind and heart, which must be emptied in order to receive new teachings. This is why in the Taoist tradition, having an "empty heart" is a privileged condition—unlike in Western culture, where emptiness means "poor"—because it allows us to welcome every new experience without prejudice or conditioning.

6. FUNDAMENTAL ACUPUNCTURE POINTS

6.1 What are acupuncture points?

The famous acupuncture points are very well-defined areas, referred to as 'points', which, when stimulated, have specific effects on certain organs or parts of the body. The points can be located in areas where there are depressions or more prominent points. In fact, with a little practice, you can learn to feel them because their density changes compared to the surrounding area. These points have been shown to have greater electrical conductivity, so stimulating them activates an impulse that reaches the brain and is then bounced back to the target organ or area. The Chinese took centuries to learn about them in depth (there are 365 points), and if after 5 millennia this practice is still held in such high regard, there is no doubt that it has much deeper roots than many scientific studies that can only boast a few decades of research.

When Chinese medicine arrived in Europe, the names of the meridians had to be codified with those of the organs, for reasons of association of ideas. In Chinese medicine, however, the meridians are named according to energy levels, an approach that is already different starting from the name. The consequence is that in the West, the points have taken on Cartesian coordinates: meridian/organ = longitude, number = latitude. In Chinese nomenclature, each point has a name that characterizes it, describing its nature or what it acts on. There are many points that refer to water and therefore act on the water element, as well as fire, or gui, spirits, and therefore influence psychic aspects, and so on. Learning the names of the points leads to a deeper understanding of them, while knowledge of the coordinates leads to a mnemonic understanding of the points.

6.2 Points and meridians

The meridian, on the other hand, is a line of electrical flow that finds a more sensitive, more effective area in the points. In fact, however, the meridian has its own identity and through it, energy passes through the points, reaches the organs, and passes from one part of the body to another, shifting and rebalancing imbalances, deficits, and energy stagnation. There are deep meridians, those treated by acupuncture, and tendinomuscular meridians, which affect a more superficial area but follow the path of the deep meridian, affecting an area rather than a point. After all, when practicing massage (shiatsu or tuina) or applying moxa, we work mainly on this type of meridian.

The main meridians are 12 pairs symmetrical to the linea alba (the central line of our body). There are also 8 extraordinary meridians: Du mai, Ren mai, Chong mai, Dai mai, Yin Qiao mai, Yang Qiao mai, Yin wei mai, Yang wei mai. We can say that these are the main meridians used in acupuncture, massage, and moxa because they are the meridians that host the points. There are also other transverse connecting meridians or internal branches that enter the organs, but to work on these types of branches, we act on specific points, so we will not go into further detail on this topic.

The important thing to know is that, according to one of the most important authors of Chinese medicine texts, Sun Si Miao, treatments should be performed on a maximum of three meridians at a time, while a skilled Chinese doctor uses a maximum of three acupuncture points in each treatment. Too many stimuli create too much information flow and disorder in the flow of Qi.

Some meridians can be combined to treat specific issues:

Du Mai: yang

Ren mai: Yin

Chong Mai: Xue (blood)

Dai Mai: upper-lower balance

Bladder: posterior muscle chain

Kidney: yin, bones, and marrow

Liver: blood and stasis or diffusion of Qi

Gallbladder: tendons and muscle strength

Pericardium: blood and diaphragm, emotions

Triple heater: energy that activates the 3 dan tian, alchemical transformation

Small intestine: purification of heat in the intestines

Heart: the Shen

Stomach: muscle mass

Spleen: the transformation of fluids

Lungs: the distribution of Qi and the immune system

Large intestine: elimination and release of waste.

Obviously, this is a simplification and an extreme summary, but it is useful for immediately directing our attention to one or a few meridians.

6.3 Key points

We will list some points that are universally recognized as fundamental or with undisputed effectiveness for certain disorders. Undoubtedly, as far as tendinomuscular meridians are concerned (and therefore those affecting motor disorders), Xi points are of great importance, especially in Yang meridians. In addition, well points and yuan points are always useful. To these we add the points that I define as fundamental because they have undisputed effectiveness in many pathologies and disorders. The treatment of points through massage or self-massage is suitable for everyone. Simply press with your thumb perpendicular to the point and knead the area, which may often be painful (typical is the LI4 or SP9 point on the left in women). Slow, deep kneading tends to "charge" the point, while faster kneading tends to discharge it. It will then be up to each individual's experience and sensitivity to understand how to treat the point.

It makes no sense to list the points in order of importance, so I will proceed according to a classification based on ease of use. We will therefore start with the 'well points'. These are located at the ends of the hands or feet, where the meridians start or end. They are usually near the nail or on the last phalanx. This makes them easy to stimulate, simply by pinching them with the index finger or thumbnail. Stimulating the well points has the function of bringing the Qi of the meridian outwards - if stimulated in dispersion, by pinching the point quickly and repeatedly. Some well points are treated by bleeding to eliminate toxins present in the meridian. Alternatively, they can be stimulated to charge the meridian if a Qi deficiency is felt, using slower and deeper pressure.

BL 67: corner of the fifth toe, purifies heat, eliminates wind from the eyes and head (treats migraines and tinnitus), helps turn the fetus if breech (with moxa)

KI1: on the sole of the foot in the depression formed by flexing the foot between the second and third metatarsals, calms the Shen, rebalances yang, treats insomnia, emotional excesses (anger, fear, madness, agitation), hot flashes during menopause, poor memory.

GB44: on the back of the fourth toe, outer nail corner, calms the Shen, purifies heat, treats dizziness, tinnitus (from liver fire), insomnia and nightmares, redness, swelling, and pain in the eyes.

LR1: on the big toe, outer nail corner (towards the second toe), calms the Shen, regulates the Qi of the lower heater, restores consciousness, alleviates pain, treats blood-related problems (in menstruation, epistaxis, hernias, and diuresis problems).

ST45: on the back of the second toe, outer nail corner, calms the Shen, purifies the heat of the meridian, restores consciousness, treats loss of consciousness, panic, insomnia, dizziness, sore throat, heat associated with pain in the face and head in general, toothache (lower arch).

SP1: on the big toe, inner nail corner, stops bleeding, restores consciousness, calms the Shen, frees the chest and rebalances the spleen, treats insomnia, sadness, excessive dreaming, dyspnea and sighing, fullness in the chest, vomiting, diarrhea, swelling in the four limbs, manic-depressive syndrome.

SI1: On the little finger of the hand, outer nail corner, purifies heat, benefits the orifices of the heart (sense organs), restores consciousness, promotes lactation, treats headaches, dizziness, conjunctivitis, epistaxis, deafness, tinnitus, oral ulcers, stroke, cough, treats the breast and chest area.

HT9: on the little finger, dorsal area, inner nail corner, helps the tongue, eyes, and throat, purifies heat, restores consciousness, calms the Shen, rebalances the Qi of the heart, treats Qi deficiency, fear, sighing, sadness, manic-depressive syndromes, eye pain, sore throat, epilepsy.

TE1: on the ring finger, outer nail corner, benefits the ears and throat, purifies the heat of the upper Jiao, promotes Qi circulation in the meridian, alleviates pain, treats fever, chills, tinnitus, deafness, headache, red eyes, dizziness, sore throat, earache.

PC9: on the middle finger, at the tip in the center, purifies heat in the heart and pericardium, eliminates external heat, treats collapse, diarrhea, vomiting, agitation, fever, restores consciousness in feverish states.

LI1: on the index finger, inner nail corner, purifies heat, relieves pain, reduces swelling, treats loss of consciousness, deafness, tinnitus, ear disorders, toothache (jaw), pain and swelling in the nasal cavity.

LU11: on the thumb, inner nail corner, restores consciousness, purifies heat, benefits the throat, treats acute swelling, congestion and pain in the throat, mumps, mania. It is one of the 13 Gui points and treats the dissociation between Hun and Po.

Let's now move on to the 4 gates, which represent a widely used protocol for energizing Qi in the four limbs and allowing excesses to be eliminated and stagnation to be moved:

LI4 - Hegu: large intestine 4, helps eliminate excess heat. Generally, the two points have a different consistency and painfulness on the two hands: the tendency is to charge the more sunken one and discharge the fuller one. It induces childbirth, alleviates pain, helps the orifices of the head, eliminates wind, toothache, sore throat, rhinitis, and headache.

LR3: Tai Chong: liver 3, is the lower gate compared to Hegu and the use of these two points together involves a dynamization of Qi between high and low and frees stasis, eliminates liver wind, subdues yang, used in headaches, frees obstructions of the head orifices.

Xi points or slit points: these are very important points because they help to unblock the meridians and are mainly used for joint, muscle, and tendon pain, so they are mainly used on the tendinomuscular meridians (therefore more superficially and through massage or moxa). They are more effective in treating yang meridians because, again with reference to the tendinomuscular meridians, they occupy a larger portion of the body and wider muscle groups. Therefore, in the explanation of the points, only the additional effects beyond the improvement of the Qi circulation of the meridian will be described, both at the energetic level (thus acting on the functions of the relevant zang-fu) and at the muscular and tendinous level.

BL63 (yang): relaxes the tendons, calms internal wind, relieves pain, treats abdominal pain, hernia, constipation, diarrhea, vomiting, and epilepsy.

KI5 (yin): regulates the conception vessel and chong mai, regulates blood flow.

GB36 (yang): alleviates pain, purifies heat, detoxifies poisons, headaches, manias, acute and painful conditions, stiffness of the neck and nape, intolerance to cold and wind.

LR6 (yin): regulates blood, disperses dampness, regulates the lower jiao, coldness in the lower limbs, numbness in the hands and feet, flaccidity of the legs.

ST34 (yang): rebalances the stomach, relieves pain, alleviates acute conditions, treats acute epigastric pain and knee disorders.

SP8 (yin): strengthens the blood, eliminates dampness, treats lack of appetite, abdominal pain and distension, edema.

SI6 (yang): relieves pain, benefits the shoulder and arm, benefits the eyes, treats pain and heaviness in the lumbar region, pain and limited mobility of the foot, weak vision, and cataracts.

HT6 (yin): calms the Shen, regulates blood, purifies yin deficiency fire, treats chest fullness, excessive worry, fear and palpitations, night sweats.

TE7 (yang): benefits the ears, treats epilepsy, tinnitus, deafness, and diffuse superficial pain (skin).

PC4 (yin): calms the Shen, purifies heat, strengthens the blood, dissolves stasis, treats insomnia, fear and terror of people, melancholy, heat hemorrhages.

LI7 (yang): calms the Shen, purifies fire and harmonizes the stomach and large intestine, purifies heat and detoxifies poisons, treats tooth and facial pain, painful nodules.

LU6 (yin): spreads lung Qi, purifies heat and moistens the lung, relieves acute conditions, treats shortness of breath, asthma, cough, yin deficiency fever, elbow, arm, and finger pain.

Yuan points are points that draw original energy from the organs, or rather, from the energy lodges. Therefore, we can see them as points that open the reservoirs of original, basal energy from that lodge and thus strengthen its functionality. They are typically located near the wrist or ankle.

BL64: calms the Shen, relaxes the tendons, eliminates wind, purifies the head and eyes, treats acute headaches, palpitations, rhinitis, visual dizziness, and cold feet.

KI3: strengthens kidney yang and tones the yin of the meridian, purifies empty heat, tones any kidney deficiency (yin, yang, and Qi), treats insomnia, poor memory, asthma, headaches, dizziness, impotence or sexual exhaustion, and cold lower limbs.

GB40: helps the circulation of liver and gallbladder Qi, alleviates pain, purifies heat and dampness in the meridian, helps the joints, treats lower limb disorders, sciatica, h l pain and cramps in the legs and hips, painful obstruction of the ankles, sighing, inability to catch one's breath, herpes zoster, gallbladder.

LR3: rebalances liver yang, eliminates wind, nourishes blood and liver yin, purifies the eyes and head, treats contractures and pain with LI4, difficulty in evacuation (urine and feces), dizziness, headache, and blurred vision.

ST42: calms the Shen, alleviates pain, promotes Qi circulation in the meridian, purifies heat in the meridian, treats ankle pain, epilepsy, fear and palpitations, mania, sadness, visions, reddened face and eyes.

SP3: rebalances Qi, tones the spleen, resolves dampness and damp-heat, treats joint and lower back pain, feverish states with fullness and oppression, vomiting, constipation, swelling of the limbs, feeling of heaviness, bone pain and edema of the limbs, undigested food in the stool.

SI4: alleviates pain, purifies heat, reduces swelling, purifies dampness-heat, treats upper limb and head disorders, tinnitus, lacrimation, jaundice, loss of taste.

HT7: calms the Shen, treats disorientation, insomnia, depression, epilepsy, poor memory, fear, restless sleep, fullness in the chest.

TE4: relaxes tendons, relieves pain, clears heat, treats pain and weakness in the wrist area.

PC7: calms the Shen, refreshes the blood, regulates the stomach and intestines, purifies heat in the heart, treats carpal tunnel syndrome, skin disorders, fever with agitation, bad breath, sighing, vomiting, sadness, insomnia, restlessness.

LI4: induces labor, helps the sense organs, eliminates wind, nourishes yang, treats febrile diseases, sneezing, sore throat, epistaxis, toothache, rhinitis, mumps, facial swelling, hemiplegia, arm pain, headache, deafness and tinnitus, eye diseases, painful atrophy of the limbs.

LU9: strengthens the lungs, transforms phlegm, regulates and harmonizes all meridians, alleviates pain, treats shortness of breath, dyspnea, asthma, cough, shortness of breath, heat in the palms, dry throat, frequent yawning, manic delirium, pain in the shoulder and supraclavicular area.

The last series of selected points are important because they are highly effective and are often used alone to resolve acute situations. Some points are repeated to focus attention on the most frequent use with which they are treated.

LI11: Quchi, relieves pain, rebalances Qi and blood, supports the immune system, used for toothache

HT7: Shenmen, calms Shen, relaxes, used for insomnia, depression, excessive worry

PC6: Neiguan, internal barrier, regulates Qi and Shen, unblocks the diagram, relieves nausea, helps with insomnia and apprehension, used for asthma and purifies heat

TE5: Waiguan, external barrier, disperses wind and heat, alleviates pain, acts on the head and ears (all disorders), toothache, and problems with the three joints of the arm: shoulder, elbow, and wrist

ST36: Zusanli, strengthens Qi, nourishes blood and Yin, purifies fire, dissolves dampness, strengthens the legs, restores consciousness, rebalances the stomach, acts on many gastrointestinal disorders

SP6: Sanyinjiao, intersection of the 3 yin: strengthens the blood, induces labor, helps the stomach and spleen, resolves dampness, regulates diuresis, tones the kidney and harmonizes the liver, acts on genital disorders and fluid stasis in general (including masses)

ST30: Qichong, assault of Qi: rebalances the lower jiao by allowing Qi to descend towards the legs

GB30: Huantiao: pain and contractures, paresthesia, dissolves wind and dampness

GB34: Yanglingquan: purifies dampness and heat from the meridian, benefits tendons and joints, sciatica, nausea, vomiting, neck and shoulder stiffness

ST40: Fenglong: purifies dampness and phlegm in the body and organs, calms the Shen, headache, agitation

ST13: Qihu, gate of Qi: reduces rebellious Qi, fullness in the chest, asthma, shortness of breath, dyspnea

CV7: Yinjiao, Yin crossing: rebalances yin in the subumbilical area and genitals

CV6: Qihai, sea of Qi: rebalances Qi, harmonizes blood, strengthens kidneys and yang, counteracts cold and prolapse (yang deficiency).

CV17: Shanzhong, center of the chest: sea point of Qi, frees the chest, treats dyspnea, cough, asthma, digestive difficulties, stomach Qi.

GV4: Mingmen, gate of life: rebalances the governing vessel, strengthens the kidneys, benefits the lumbar area, purifies heat, treats dizziness, tinnitus, epilepsy, rectal prolapse, hemorrhoids.

GV14: Dazhui, great vertebra: sea point of Qi, calms and expels wind, purifies heat, treats emptiness, fever and chills, sore throat, night sweats, lack of strength, epilepsy, neck disorder (moxa recommended).

GV20: Baihui, hundred meetings: sea point of the marrow, calms wind and Shen, subdues and raises yang, benefits the head and sense organs, treats loss of consciousness, prolapse and symptoms of kidney yang deficiency, poor memory, disorientation, sadness with suicidal thoughts, stroke, visual disturbances, tinnitus, headache, dizziness.

Yintang: extra-meridian point, between the eyebrows: calms the Shen, subdues wind, relieves pain, treats insomnia, anxiety and agitation, relieves headaches and all discomfort resulting from nasal congestion.

6.4. Meridian maps

Below are maps of the main meridians. The purpose is to give an idea of their path in order to have an idea of the path of the tendinomuscular meridians, a useful notion for acting through gymnastic exercises, strengthening, or stretching where there is a need to work on specific meridians based on the indications that our body gives us, whether it is an indication of the state of health of the muscles or an indication of the state of health of the organs.

Urinary Bladder (BL)

Bladder Meridian (BL)

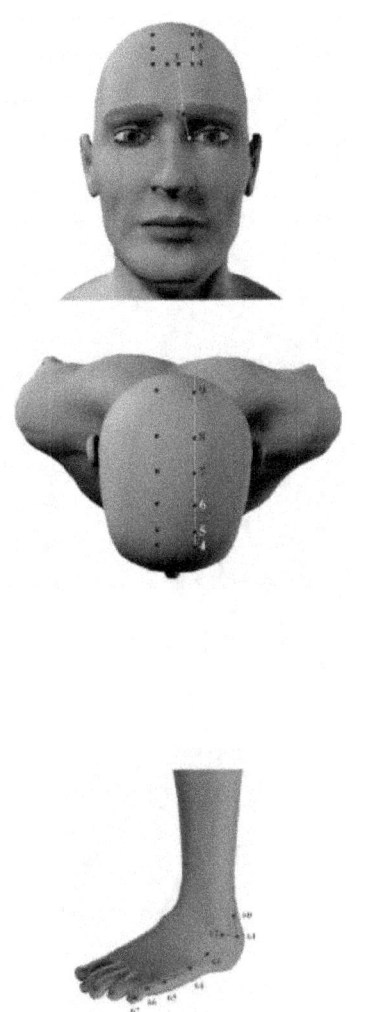

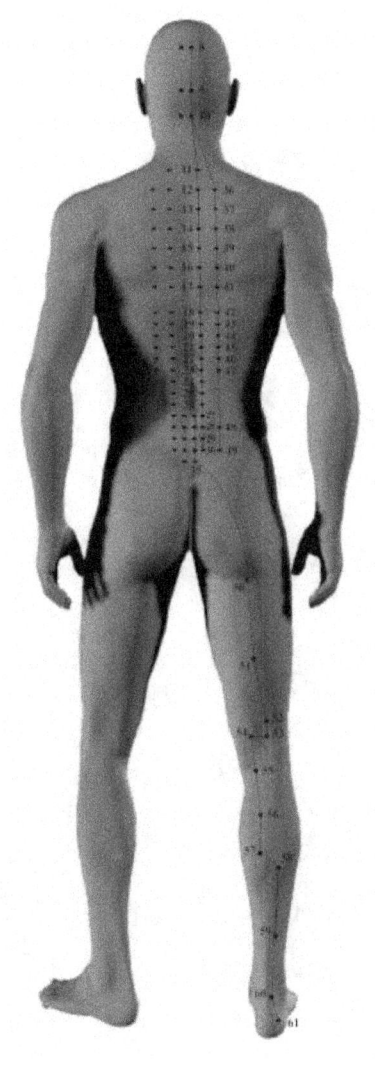

Kidney (KI)

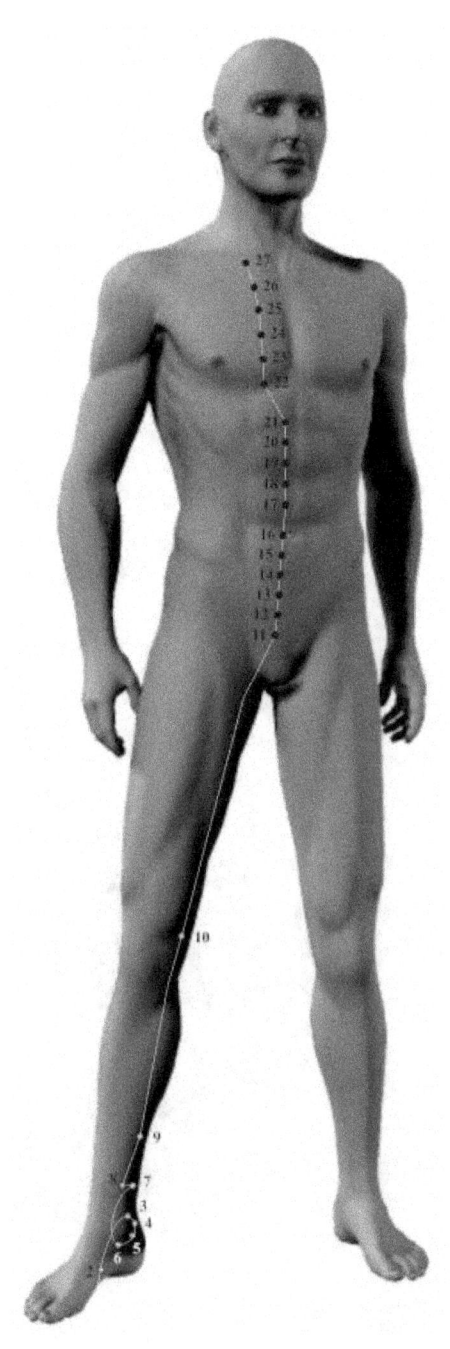

Gallbladder (GB)

105

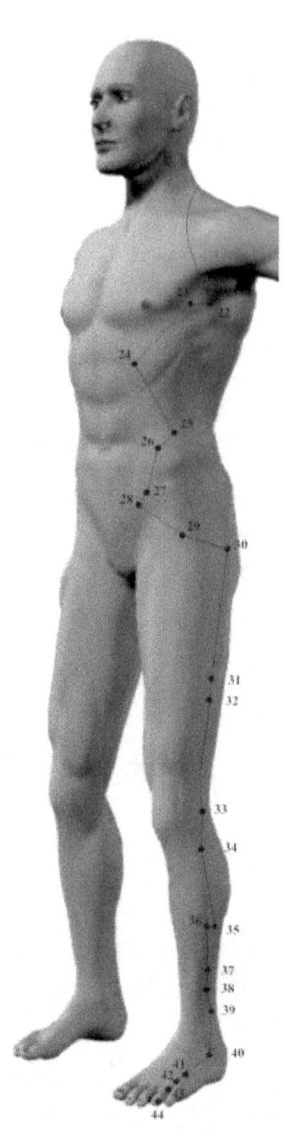

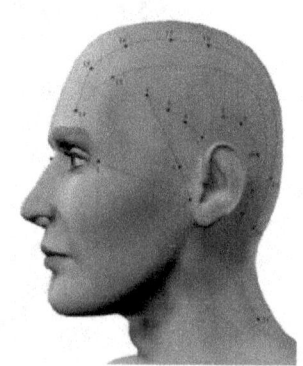

Liver (LR)

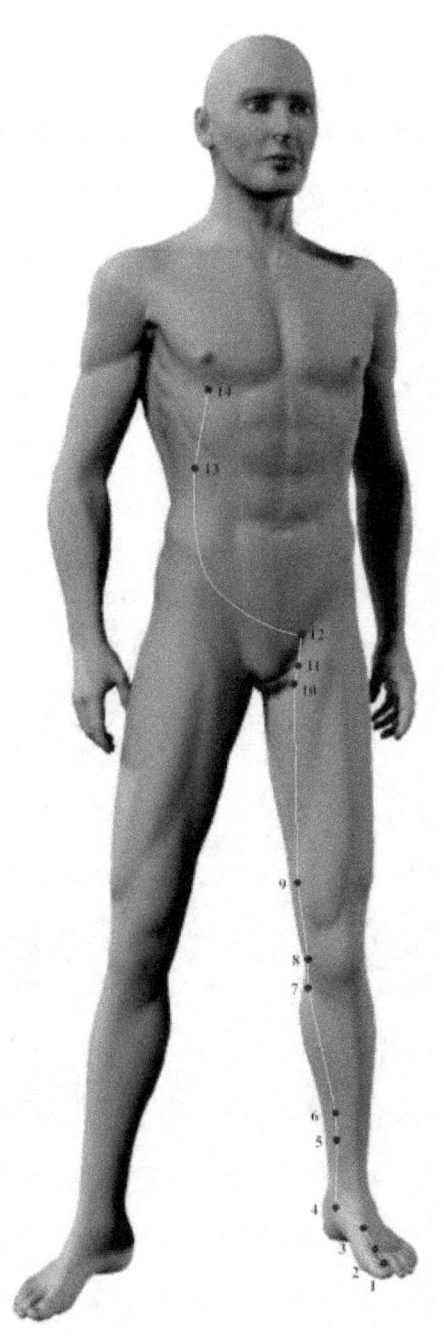

Stomach (ST)

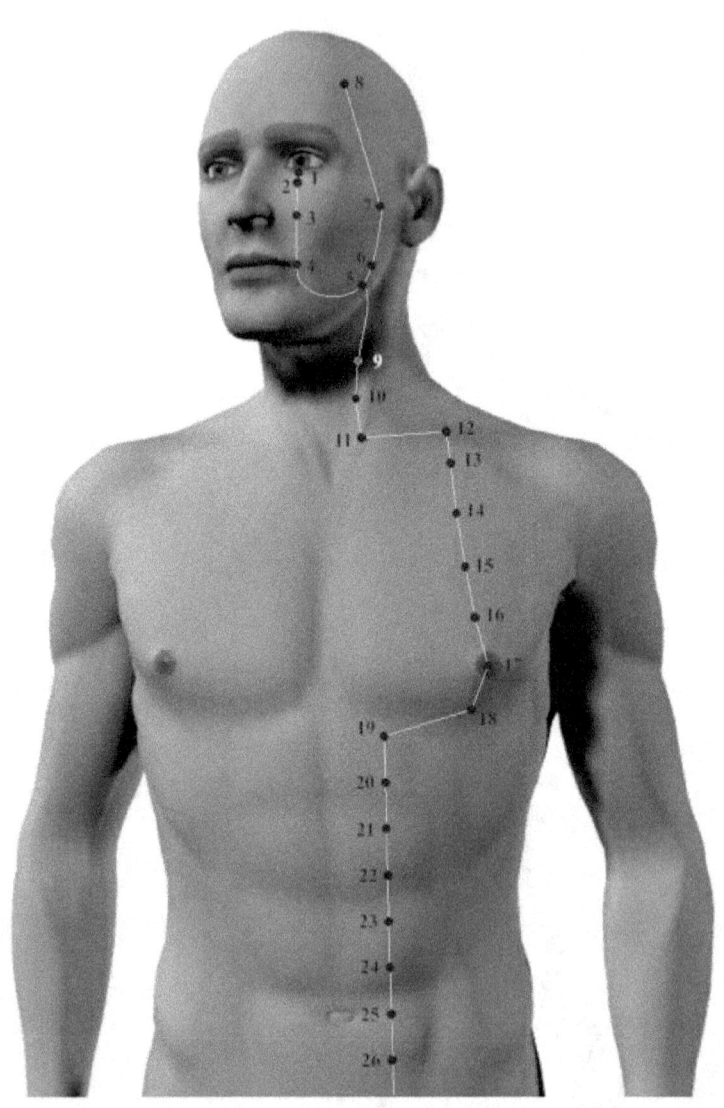

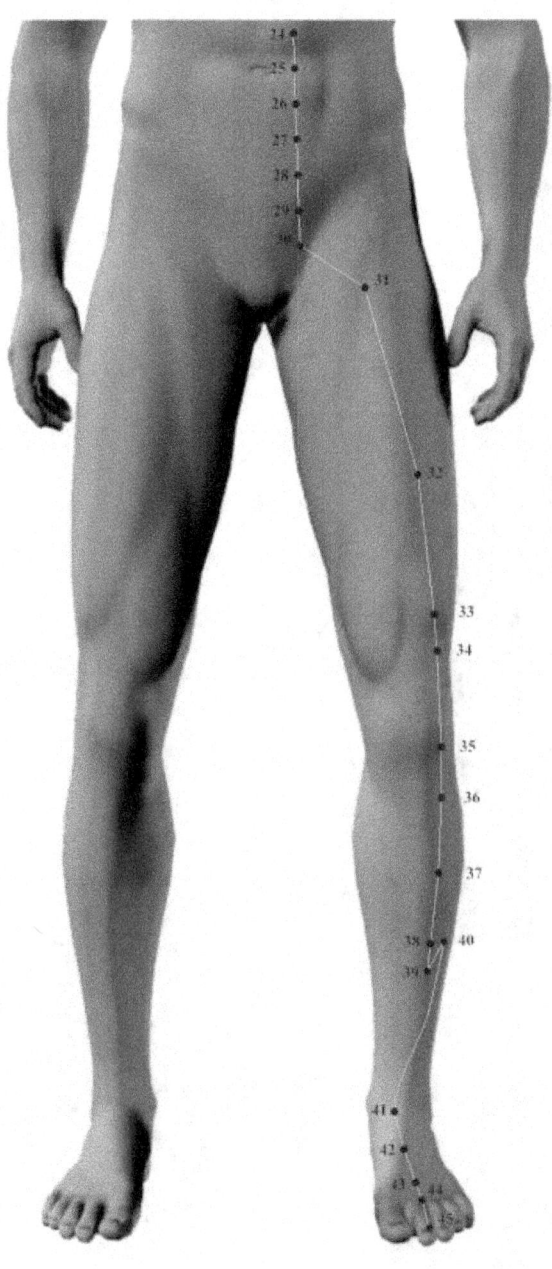

Spleen Pancreas (SP)

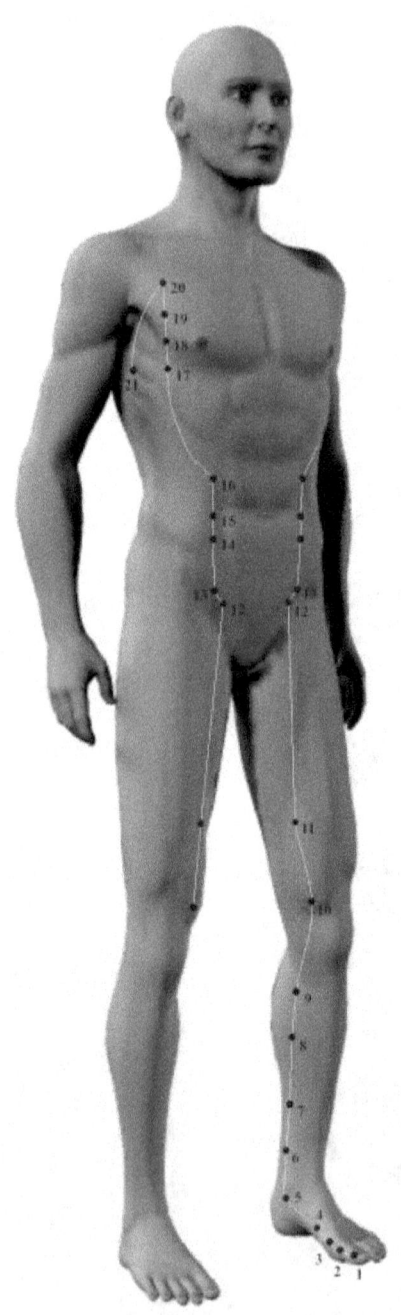

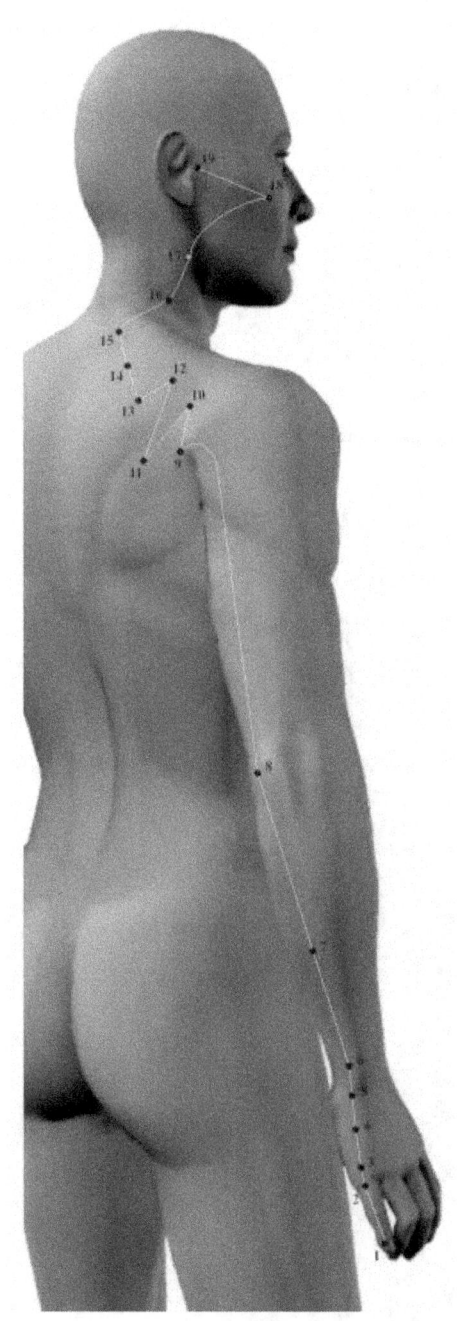

Small intestine (SI)

Heart (HT)

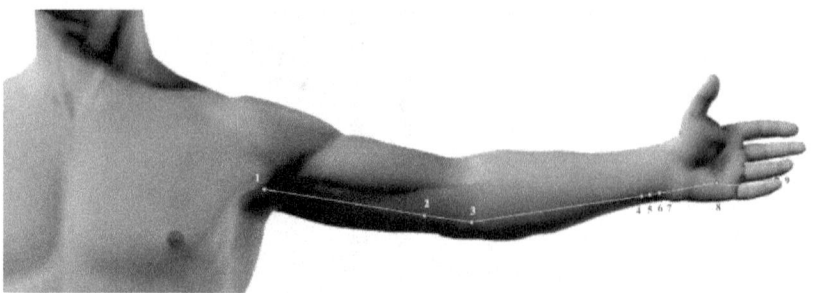

Triple heater (TE)

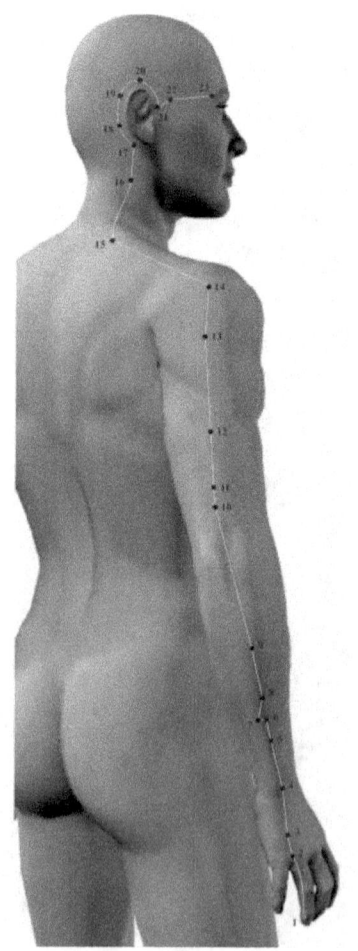

Pericardium (PC)

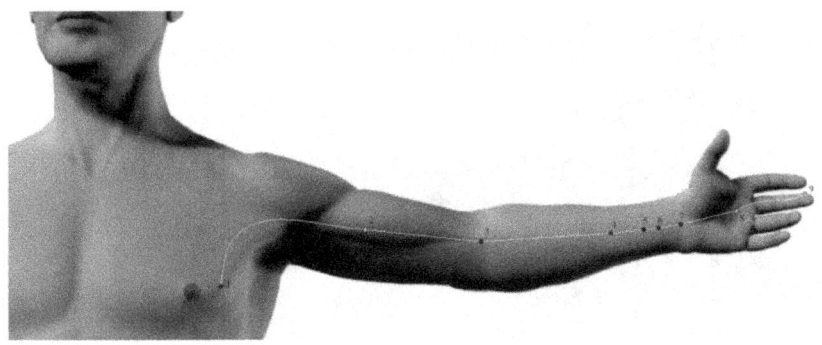

Large intestine (LI)

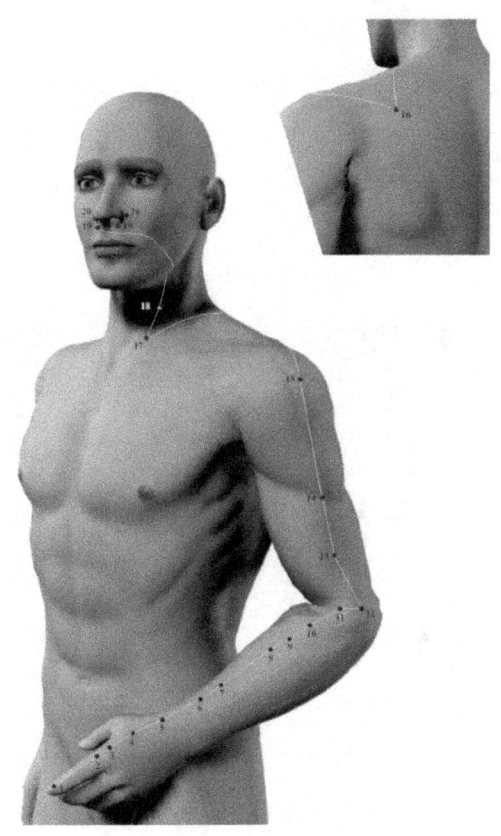

113

Lung (LU)

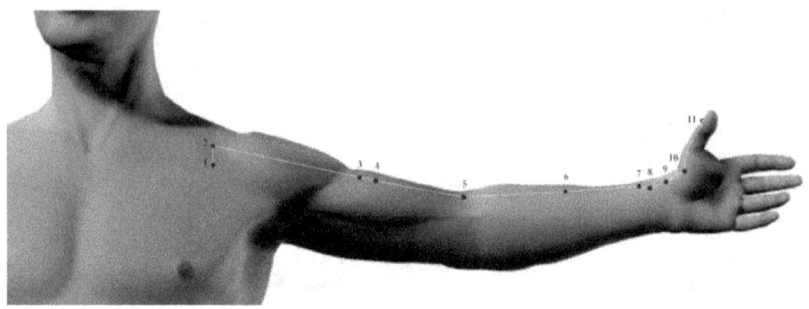

Governor Vessel – Du mai

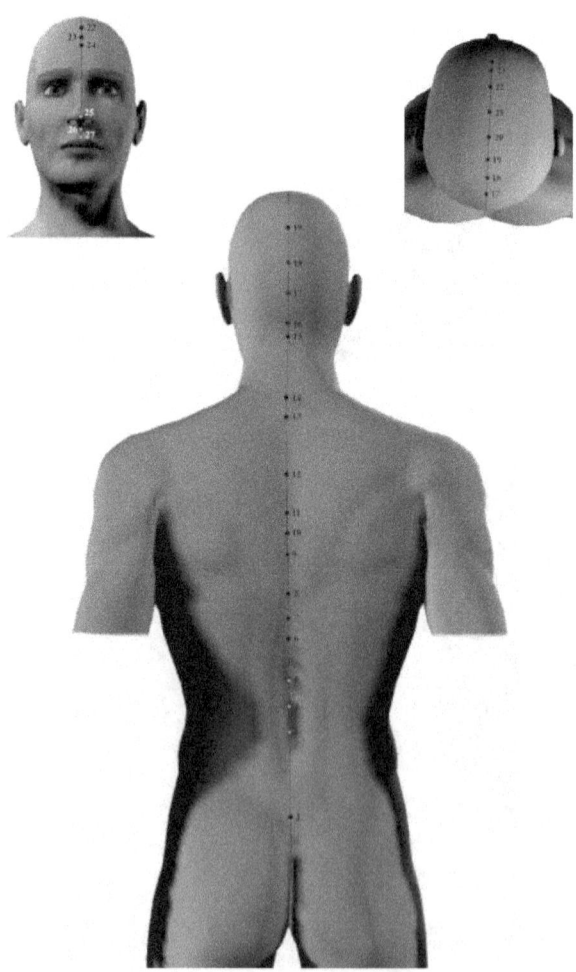

Conception Vessel – Ren mai

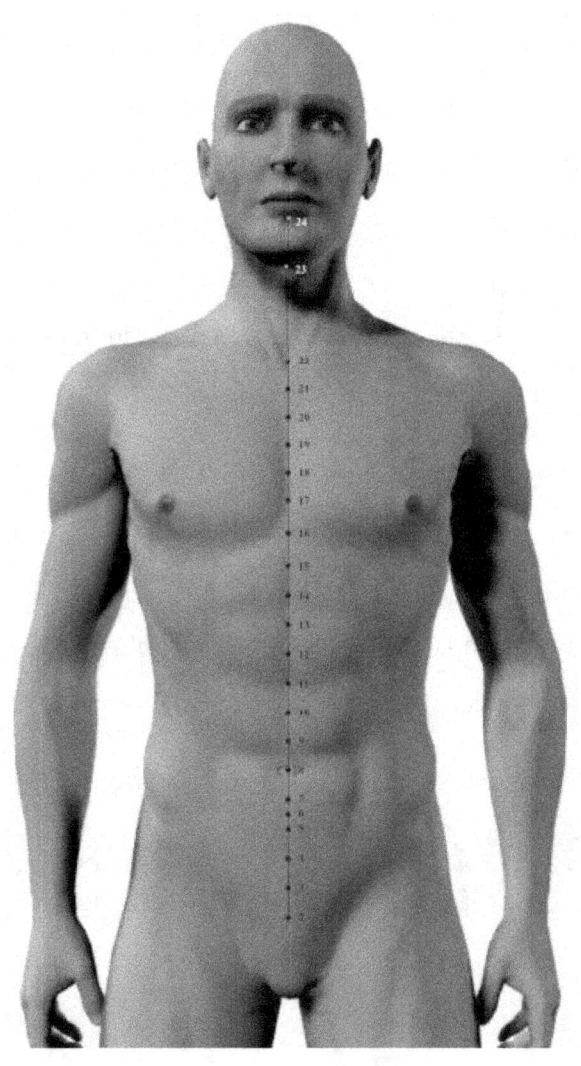

7. THE BODY AND MOVEMENT

As mentioned above, Chinese medicine is based on five pillars: acupuncture, massage, dietetics, herbal medicine, and Qigong. Only the latter is a practice where the individual is totally responsible for themselves because they do not receive or seek external input but must take action personally and feel what happens when they practice Qigong.

At this stage, referring to the San Bao, we will mainly talk about Qi, as it represents the most controllable energy element and the one on which the individual can work the most, while Jing is a hereditary factor and Shen is a more mental/psychological factor, so we can say that it 'comes after training the body'.

7.1 The Role of Movement in Health and Well-being

The basic principle for health in the tradition of Chinese medicine is that health is present if Qi flows freely. Qi flows freely if the blood flows well. It is said that Qi is the rider of blood. Therefore, Qi pushes the blood, and if blood circulation is good in terms of frequency and intensity, it means that Qi is good and is pushing the blood correctly. Where Qi is scarce, stagnation can occur, not only of blood but also of other fluids (Jin ye). Where Qi flows freely, the muscles contract and relax in an elastic, flexible, and vigorous manner. When contractures form, Qi no longer flows well, the muscle locks up and no longer allows Qi to pass through, and consequently, neither does blood. In these cases, hematomas or edema may form. Therefore, stretching is necessary to release the blockage. When you have a strain or, worse still, a muscle tear, there is an interruption in the structure and Qi can no longer flow, making the situation even more serious. In fact, as mentioned, every 'fracture' of tissue (whether bone, tendon, or muscle) creates an interruption and Qi can no longer flow. During the healing phase, Qi gradually resumes its usual pathways and flow is restored, but this does not always happen completely. In other words, the condition prior to the trauma is not always restored. On a superficial level, this situation is evident when scars appear, but scars can also be deep. Each scar represents a barrier to the flow of Qi, which, in most cases, is resolved by restoring the flow of Qi to over 90%. However, in some cases, toxic scars (purple, painful, nodular, or fibrous) occur. These must be treated because, in addition to preventing the flow of Qi, they keep the area and the meridian in a state of perpetual inflammation, which weakens and sometimes limits mobility, albeit minimally. There have been cases where, after a trauma resulting in scarring, people have begun to suffer from neck pain, migraines, stiff neck, and frozen shoulder.

You see, when a problem arises on a physical level, whether visible or not, the consequence is that Qi encounters an obstacle or can no longer find its way. By working on these obstacles, i.e., preventing obstacles or interruptions from forming and thus keeping our channels operational and free, we will create preferential pathways for our Qi. It is true that accidents can occur that can injure us in some way and thus block our Qi, but it is more likely that such a situation will occur in a body that has not trained its Qi to flow freely.

The consequences of good Qi flow, to mention just a few of the benefits, are a better cardiovascular system (in terms of frequency, power, recovery, blood pressure), a better cardiorespiratory system (better blood oxygenation, slower and deeper breathing with greater elimination of toxins, better management of anxiety and situations of 'air hunger' thanks to breath control), a better musculoskeletal structure (greater bone density, greater joint flexibility, greater strength thanks to the ability of the tendons to contract, greater resistance to exertion), and so on.

Movement also has benefits for the mind. In fact, it has been shown that engaging in exercises that require r coordination, and a sufficient amount of effort allows us to focus on what we are doing and thus temporarily free ourselves from thoughts, worries, and fears: by engaging in something, without the need to reach the competitive trance state that endurance athletes enjoy so much but which has an erosive effect on muscles and joints (compensated for with supplements), we can enter a mental state similar to meditation. It may be that the heart rate accelerates due to greater physical effort, but brain waves slow down, bringing us to the Alpha frequency. As we continue with the practice, we can even reach a Theta brain wave frequency, which means activating the parasympathetic system, i.e., cell regeneration, as when we sleep, but also strengthening and supporting the immune system.

The big difference between activities that consume and those that 'nourish' is precisely this: above a certain threshold, the structure is consumed and even at the cerebral level, we remain at a level of mental excitement (our software) so that the recovery and regeneration program is never started: it is as if we set the computer without energy saving and even if we are not doing any work, the battery is consumed.

As mentioned in the previous chapter, once the Qi is depleted, we move on to consuming Jing. When our body has exhausted its sugar reserves, it draws energy from the muscles. If the movement we perform is not perfect, the muscle gradually loses strength, coordination, and perfection in its execution as it is consumed, forcing the joints and tendons, which in these cases can even lead to injury.

Have you ever taken a long, long walk in the mountains? Have you noticed that when you can't take it anymore, even if you're going downhill, you bump your feet more frequently against rocks or other obstacles? This is a sign that your muscles are so tired that you are losing coordination in your movements and you are placing your feet badly or not lifting them high enough... When we lose control due to fatigue, it doesn't take much (a rolling stone, a protruding root...) to twist an ankle or knee... and thus incur more or less serious damage.

So the principle for a healthy body is: move according to your abilities, availability, aptitudes, and pleasure. Yes, because we don't have to do gymnastics with equipment if we don't like it. We don't have to do yoga because all my friends do it and say it's great. I don't have to go to the pool because the doctor said so... Of course, there are various activities that are recommended for health reasons, but if they require technical skills and a r awareness of the body's movements, and we don't have these and there is no one to supervise us, we could cause even more damage to our bodies. And if we decide to practice an activity that we don't like but have been "convinced" to practice, we can be absolutely certain that we will harm our bodies because the execution of the movement will be conditioned by a lack of enthusiasm and therefore a lack of attention and a lack of mental Qi in what we are doing.

Of course, because the emotional aspect is important in any activity: whether it's work, spending time with family, playing a game of tennis, watching a movie, or reading a book. If the mind is not present, we are not present. Or rather, if the mind wants to be elsewhere, it will also sabotage the body.

Above all, the mind must be present in what we are about to do: body, soul, and spirit (mind) must be aligned and consistent so that the body moves correctly and effectively, the soul is emotionally involved and finds pleasure in what it does, and the mind has a perception of space, time, and the execution of what is being done. On the contrary: an untrained person or one without technical skills will have physical limitations; a person who does not want to do or actually despises that type of activity will not put in the right energy or will not put it in at all and will have limitations in getting excited and activating the emotional and h l aspects of the activity. Finally, a person who is drunk or does not know the rules or does not understand how to optimize their energy resources and immediately uses up all their fuel will have limitations from a mental and rational point of view.

For example, if we are about to go climbing and we think that our boss has denied us the raise we hoped for... we may never be able to get past the first challenging 'pitch', even if we have done it before. But there are a thousand other examples that I won't mention here. Therefore, it is essential to devote ourselves to an activity that we enjoy, that we are passionate about, that is not a commitment or a duty but a space in the week that we look forward to and can't wait to repeat as soon as possible. Of course, there are days when we would like to switch off and have no obligations, and this is where awareness of what we do and, above all, the effects it has on us (body, soul, and spirit) comes into play: if I know that after a workout I feel more toned, energetic, and cheerful... even if the day has been terrible, I will try to train because the effect will be all the more positive. This is where the concept of DISCIPLINE comes in, which in just a few years has been lost as a principle.

Successful athletes, but also musicians, researchers, and artisans, must devote enormous amounts of time, resources, and energy to achieve successful results. To do so, they must adopt a mental approach of determination and discipline: establishing rules, limits, goals, and methods to make their efforts profitable.

Doing something badly takes the same amount of time (and perhaps the same amount of energy) as doing it well. The only difference is that in the first case, we will have to redo it or someone else will have to do it for us (I always think of this when I see trash left on the street near a trash can: to do the same thing—throw away the trash—it would have been enough to take a few more steps or drop it a moment earlier or later, but inside the trash can).

As I said before, however, discipline does not become a nuisance if there is pleasure in what you do or if there are goals you want to achieve through that activity. Sometimes the end justifies the means, but as a Taoist adage says: it is not the destination but the journey that enriches us with experience.

If we read this from a Taoist perspective, the coherence of the three centers mentioned above can be compared to the San Bao, which must also be in harmony. What does this mean? It means that my Jing, my Qi, and my Shen must be "favorable" to the activity I decide to do.

Jing as physical structure, predisposition to perform that activity.

Qi as energy, as a resource (time is also a resource) to be able to do it.

Shen, as pleasure, interest, stimulus, willingness to do it.

You see? Balance and harmony are never just a matter of one factor, but of all three factors: body (Jing), energy (Qi), and spirit (Shen), which is very similar to the triptych of other disciplines that see the individual as composed of "body, soul, and spirit." In fact, in Chinese medicine, "energy" should be replaced with "soul," because what enlivens is precisely what animates, but this is not the place to get into such hair-splitting arguments.

7.2 Exercises to stimulate the meridians

Stimulating the meridians actually means allowing Qi to flow freely, smoothly, and vigorously. Always, in whatever activity we do.

Breathing

To introduce this topic, I will use one of the typical—albeit incomplete—translations of the word Qi: breath. Many have translated the concept of Qi with a noun from our vocabulary. Let me open a parenthesis: words in Chinese are often a concept and not just a finished noun. Of course, a horse is a horse, but Qi is not just breath, just as Xue is not just blood, Shen is not just spirit, and so on.

Returning to breath: the lung is the minister of Qi, the one who spreads it throughout every part of the body, pushing it everywhere... just as it pushes the air to be expelled outwards. In fact, the lung's ' ' is active during exhalation, while during inhalation, according to Chinese physiology, it is the kidney that activates this action and holds the breath. This is why breathing is essential for energy to flow through the meridians and why all Eastern disciplines, which are defined as holistic but which I prefer to define as 'energetic' when it comes to physical practices, attach great importance to breathing.

Breathing should be calm, deep, long, without forcing, and will gradually become slower, deeper, and lighter: in this way, Qi is not pushed violently into the body and if it encounters an obstacle (contracture, edema, scar), it can avoid it without stopping: a bit like if we spray a hose against a perforated wall, the result will be that little water will pass through the wall. However, if we use several jets with a short range but directed at the holes, we will be able to get almost all the water through the wall. Breathing is also related to heart rate: in fact, for every breath we take, our heart beats 4-5 times. This means that, on average, an adult takes 15-16 breaths per minute. When we speed up our breathing, our heart rate also increases, but we have all noticed this when doing any kind of physical exercise.

But is it breathing that affects heart rate, or is it heart rate that accelerates breathing rate to bring in more oxygen? It is breathing that affects heart rate because we can influence our breathing and, as a result, the heart will also harmonize with our breathing. This is why training our breathing also makes our cardiovascular system more efficient. Furthermore, there is no doubt that keeping a calm heart improves our lives, both emotionally and physically: according to the Chinese, we have 4 billion heartbeats at our disposal. This means that if we stress our heart physically or emotionally, this will increase our heart rate and reduce its remaining life. This is not just a question of physical activity or sport, but also of emotions. In fact, if we think of someone who suffers from anxiety attacks, we will see a person with shallow, rapid breathing and an involuntary and unmotivated acceleration of the heartbeat. Whether they like it or not, these people put their hearts under stress, even though they are not doing any physically demanding activity that requires greater diffusion of Qi. In fact, when we exert ourselves, more Qi needs to circulate in the body, as well as more Xue (which is pushed by Qi) to nourish the muscles and organs. Emotional stress, on the other hand, does not require any additional Qi beyond the basal metabolic rate, but it accelerates the heart rate and the Qi is either dispersed or trapped.

Therefore, breathing deeply and bringing air below the navel helps to spread Qi and Xue throughout the body. Seven or eight very deep breaths are enough to realize this: the immediate effects are a sense of relaxation, a better perception of oneself and one's tensions, improved blood circulation confirmed by tingling near or upstream of the tensions, and warming of the extremities. Thanks to the lungs, we have pushed our Qi into all the energy meridians and, through the blood, we have nourished and warmed all parts of the body.

Finally, if we think about it, breathing allows us to 'take' an immaterial substance and act on matter: by entering our lungs and pushing deep into the abdomen, or by performing expansion and contraction movements, thanks to simple breathing we act mechanically on our organs and muscles. For example, if we bend our torso sideways with one arm raised and try to inhale deeply, we will feel greater tension in the intercostal area, thus exerting an important pneumatic effect, which allows us to stretch the fasciae without any physical effort.

Posture:

Secondly, we can actively stimulate the meridians by performing specific exercises that can affect individual meridians (typical of Qi gong practice) or through more complex and articulated movements that affect all meridians and are representative of applications of various movements in martial arts (Taiji and other forms of Kung fu). Personally, I believe that the path should be approached progressively, starting with simple, isolated, and repeated Qi gong movements, which are useful for acquiring the characteristics of water movement, long and deep breathing, joint mobility, and Qi support in the various energy centers, thus with a more internal purpose, and then moving on to more complex practices with a more external purpose, such as working in pairs, martial applications, form development, and so on. It's a bit like deciding to write a book: first you learn the letters and words of a language, and then you can write paragraphs, chapters, and so on.

The intensity of the practice is a purely Western and, I would say, modern issue. Qi gong originated in China to strengthen people (mainly farmers) who did hard, tiring, and exhausting work and needed to use gentler practices to get back on track, remove ailments and discomforts, recover their energy, support their organs in storing energy, and regenerate their exhausted bodies and minds. That was in the past. In the modern era, where we practice sports to compensate for the excess food we eat and to shake off the sedentary lifestyle of the vast majority of our jobs, Qi gong would seem anachronistic and a thing for old people, because it is for those who have little energy to consume.

Energy is consumed continuously, and in reality, we should use only what we need. If we think we have surplus energy, it is because we either eat too much or our work takes up too little energy, and so we have to vent it. But in reality, we could convert that energy into many other activities without necessarily consuming it physically, but no one has ever taught us this, and in reality, the economy needs consumption: consumption of food, consumption of activities, consumption of painkillers, consumption of supplements because the food we eat is caloric but not very nutritious, not very alive, with little Jing. Exercise to maintain health or to keep our bodies toned and strong should not exhaust us. Excessive consumption of Qi combined with a poor intake of nutritious Qi (food and healthy air) results in a depletion of Jing to sustain the body, causing wear and tear on muscles, joints, marrow, and so on. When we sweat a lot and do not properly replenish lost fluids and salts, we are dispersing too much Qi.

Our body has a program with an emotional memory. If it happens to suffer from a lack of water or food in a given situation, it will try to create reserves so as not to find itself in the same situation again. So not drinking during strenuous physical activity and then drinking a liter and a half of water when I'm done only creates a memory in the body and a desire to create reserves so as not to find itself in deficit. After all, what would we do if there were a period of drought? Once the event is over, we would equip ourselves with tanks to collect and dispense rainwater so as not to risk running out. So when we put our bodies under excessive stress and/or without the proper replenishment of the Yin part, the body defends itself and retains it. Then, perhaps for aesthetic reasons, we will take draining substances, or we will intensify our exercises because we will have lost definition.

The result is that we inflame our bodies. We are extremely attracted to Yang, and the more we feed it, the more we need it. It is dopamine, it is compulsiveness, it is the continuous desire stimulated by continuous external inputs that actually cause us to enter a loop and a mechanicality of our existence that we sometimes lose awareness of. Just ask yourself: how much do I like doing this? How much does it make me feel good? Is it a commitment or a pleasure? Am I willing to not do it if I don't feel well for a few days, or am I addicted/enslaved to the situation so that I can't get out of the loop? How much does it matter to me compared to how much it matters that I show it to others? There are certain practices that lead to a sort of trance (running, dancing, climbing) that often help us enter other levels of consciousness, so that we break out of automatism or, rather, by forcing automatism to such an extent that we break through the fabric and enter a dimension where the purely physical part disappears. The important thing, even in those cases, is to ask yourself: am I willing to leave things half done if I don't feel like continuing? Am I willing to preserve myself even if it means missing the final goal? Respect for ourselves and the body that houses us is fundamental, and our meridians or the spiritual aspects that inhabit us know this and sooner or later tell us so.

In Qigong and Taiji, for example, the right level of intensity is reached when a light dew of sweat forms on the body. Not too much, because when you sweat a lot, Qi is dispersed and winds could enter through the open pores, making us sick (we all know that wearing sweaty clothes in the cold or wind puts us at risk of colds, muscle pain, or rheumatism). Breathing will only be slightly faster but, above all, it will be deeper: you will be able to act on the diaphragm, which in more stressed people is at risk of becoming blocked, causing shallow breathing. When we unblock the diaphragm, breathing deepens, respiratory and heart rates slow down, there is a greater and better supply of oxygen, and by breathing more deeply, the diaphragm lowers and allows the organs and viscera of the abdomen to be massaged, improving peristalsis and the elimination of waste and h l elements. The skin takes on a more vibrant color because it is better supplied with blood. Muscles will be more toned and less rigid, and more elastic thanks to the contraction and relaxation achieved through various movements, which will never attempt to reach 100% muscle capacity. Strength can be trained using additional weights once you have acquired familiarity and dexterity in the movements, but what matters is to work the muscles and tendons in their entirety, with constant intensity and without jerks or tugs, because doing so only trains reactive strength but not holding strength and, worse still, does not train coordination and posture. Posture does not only refer to the posture of the body but also to the optimal positioning of body segments in order to perform a movement with maximum efficiency (energy saving) and effectiveness (best result). It is not just a question of economy but also of training the body to perform the best movement that could be useful in particular conditions, perhaps even at work. If, for example, we learn to lift a weight in the optimal way, loading it onto our legs, keeping our spine aligned thanks to abdominal support, we unload the weight we are supporting with our hands by connecting our shoulder blades and in this way unloading better onto our spine and legs, we will be able to be more effective, managing to lift an unexpected weight or even just avoiding hurting our back, knees, neck, and so on.

Attention to the details of the movement becomes the extra element, but this is learned through practice because by emulating those who teach us the movement and feeling what works and what doesn't, we will gain the experience that will enable us to move tomorrow, strong as a tiger and light as a crane.

The meridians are correctly stimulated when there is no excessive effort, when the position and movement assumed is "comfortable" because if there is discomfort or pain, the difficult passage of Qi is intrinsic. There are movements that may seem uncomfortable but, on reflection, relieve tension and release it after a few repetitions: at that point, there was a blockage of Qi that struggled to pass but then overcame the obstacle and improved the condition. The meridians do not like to lose the Yin part through excessive sweating; the Qi in the tendinomuscular meridians is more superficial and it is the weiQi that has a 28-minute circulation along all the meridians, so it appreciates a phase of greater intensity and then relaxation, like the movement of a wave.

All this while assuming a correct (efficient and effective) posture/positioning, one of verticality, because man is the antenna that connects heaven to earth. We have thus arrived at the second fundamental principle for correct kinetic practice or sports , if you will: posture. After breathing, this element becomes very important, both because we keep our energy meridians and muscle groups relaxed and in "order," and because correct posture leads to greater proprioception of oneself and one's movements, thereby improving balance, coordination, and mastery in the use of the body and limbs in space: we can therefore become more skilled and capable of performing even complex, new, and unusual movements without great difficulty.

I happened to see a tennis player hitting balls with great ease and noticed taiji movements in his movements. I asked him if he practiced any Chinese gymnastics or martial arts techniques and he said no. I had him do some simple exercises where it was important to rotate the body on the central axis and shift weight from one foot to the other, and he succeeded admirably, considering it was his first experience. Similarly, I asked to play with him, and although I did not have much experience in tennis, I immediately learned some essential elements necessary to use the body well in the practice of that sport. Technically, I had to correct many things: grip, point of impact with the ball, opening moment, but the dynamics of the body were correct, and this allowed me to accelerate the learning period for that sport. It was as if 50% of the work had already been done. And this argument is replicable in many sports or physical activities. So we call posture what is awareness of one's own body, in quantitative and qualitative terms, especially meaning awareness of one's own body in space, both statically and dynamically.

Presence

I can drive and talk on the phone. I can eat while watching a movie. I can listen to an audiobook while taking a walk. But what happens if I get angry with the person I'm talking to on the phone? What happens if I chew a clove of garlic while watching the movie? What happens if I have to jump over a stream while listening to the audiobook? What will probably happen is that I won't notice a pedestrian about to cross at the crosswalk or a traffic light that has just turned red; I won't notice a detail in a scene because the unpleasant taste of garlic will have disgusted me; I'll miss the last 10-15 seconds of the audiobook because I'll have focused all my attention on finding a safe foothold and landing spot to cross the stream.

This is not an undesirable condition, mind you, but it is certainly one that we should try to avoid, especially when performing certain activities. I doubt that a surgeon would leave their cell phone on and be distracted by a message while operating. They would put it on airplane mode and then deal with it later. I doubt that a chef would leave the stove while cooking if they had doubts about whether they had locked the car.

When performing certain activities, each of us knows, or should know, that we must devote at least 95% of our attention to what we are doing. Because we want to do it well, we don't want to have to do it again, for any other good reason that comes to mind, but basically the approach we should take is one of presence, attention, and dedication. Multitasking is a joke of the modern age that has led us all to do many things superficially. Excellence, on the other hand, stands out because when you devote yourself to an activity, you do so with total presence. So even when doing exercises on the meridians and on your body, you should try to be aware of your breathing and posture (previous points), but not only that: you should avoid getting caught up in the activities of the day, the things you have to do next, or the pizza with friends the next day. In short: I devote an hour of my time to doing one thing and I must not waste energy by focusing my attention on something else that I cannot follow or develop in the meantime and which consequently causes me to perform an activity poorly. Now I am talking about exercise and physical activity, but the same applies to other situations: while I am enjoying a good pizza, I must not think about why that exercise did not go well. The answer probably lies in the fact that when I was doing that exercise, I was thinking about what pizza I wanted to eat...

I decide to devote time to taking care of my body, and that's what I do. Other activities will be done when the time is right. Being centered in the here and now is not a slogan; it is a fundamental principle of self-discipline for doing a good job, but over time it will allow us to refine our senses and feel if our meridians are well stretched, if the Qi is flowing well, if our breath reaches the tips of our hands, feet, and hair: being in ourselves and in what we are doing allows us to have a complete view of our body, physically, energetically, and emotionally.

When we align our breath, posture, and presence, our energy centers are aligned: posture (Jing and lower dantian), breath (Qi and middle dantian), presence (Shen and upper dantian), and then we are well disposed to a more effective, complete, and constructive practice for our being. And when we learn to do this in a discipline or activity (sport in this case), we learn to transfer it to everything we do: work, cooking, rest, social relationships. When the gym trains the body, energy, and spirit, a gym is enough; it is then up to us to apply it in various situations.

7.3 Exercises to stretch the meridians

We should think of our meridian system as the cloth on a pool table: if the cloth is well stretched, the balls roll perfectly. The balls are our Qi. Keep our cloth well stretched and the Qi will flow perfectly.

This does not mean that we should only do stretching exercises, because that would only stretch the cloth and, in the long run, it would become loose. Instead, we need to alternate between strengthening, holding, and stretching exercises. All this with particular attention to the tendinomuscular meridians, first and foremost, and to the deep muscles of the chest and abdomen, secondarily, but not in order of importance, but in terms of approach and methodology.

There are many stretching exercises and specific exercises for the meridians, and many books deal with the subject. But when stretching the meridians, you need to add some elements compared to "classic" stretching: work on long muscle groups or multiple muscle groups, while one muscle group tends to stretch, there must be another muscle group, or multiple muscle groups, that are working in contraction and holding. You must not let the body think that stretching means relaxation. It must be a stretching of one part while another is actively working; it can also be defined as power stretching.

For example: in the sun salutation in the triangle or dog position, the posterior muscle group is stretched, but at the same time the deltoids, dorsal and abdominal muscles are contracting and holding. It is therefore important to alternate between stretching and contracting so as not to lose muscle and tendon tone. While it is true that muscles must be elastic, they must also have their own strength, which comes from the ability to tense and contract the muscle. Dancers and gymnasts are a good example of this: they represent perfection in terms of body, movement, and control: flexibility and tension.

I will not go through the stretching exercises for the meridians, but I will indicate which areas are affected by the individual meridians:

Bladder: posterior fascia, from the nape of the neck to the heels, affecting the paravertebral muscles. This is the fascia that rests on the ground when we lie on our backs. Bending over to touch your feet is the most typical exercise affecting this meridian.

Kidneys: inner leg, from the foot to the groin (including the arch of the foot), and front of the chest to the collarbone, on the side of the linea alba. Butterfly legs, with the soles of the feet resting on top of each other.

Stomach: front of the body, from the back of the foot to the face. The area in contact with the ground when we lie on our stomach.

Cobra pose, for example. It is also important to stretch the neck muscles, the sternocleidomastoid.

Spleen: inner thighs in a more medial position than the kidneys and abdominal area: sitting with legs bent, one knee inwards and the other outwards, then twist the torso.

Large intestine: In the prone position, it is the part of the arm in contact with the ground, resting the index fingers on the ground, reaching up to the nose, also involving the sternocleidomastoid muscle.

Lungs: affects the medial inner part of the arm, starting from the thumb and reaching the intersection of the pectoral muscle with the shoulder: open the arm, bringing the thumb backwards.

Gallbladder: outer lateral fascia of the body, from the temples to the feet. Anything that twists the torso and hip area is beneficial to this fascia. Sitting with one ankle resting on the knee, try to stretch the gluteal area.

Liver: again, the inner side of the legs, feet in a butterfly position or resting elbows and knees on the ground, try to spread your legs, stretching the groin area.

Small intestine: outer area of the arm starting from the little finger, up to the ear, passing through the shoulder blade area, which is the most important area. I grab one elbow (whose arm remains extended) and bring it close to my chest, feeling the deltoid and shoulder blade area stretch well.

Heart: outer area of the arm, again starting from the little finger but involving the inner side that connects the little finger to the armpit. I grasp the little finger and bring the arm above my head, bending the elbow, and stretch the armpit and humerus area.

Triple heater: outer area of the arm, the part that touches a wall when I lean on it with the back of my hand. I stretch out one arm, grasp the back of my hand with one hand, and bend my wrist, stretching the outer muscles of the forearm.

Pericardium: inner arm up to the chest. Opposite position to the triple heater: I extend one arm, grasp my hand and bend my wrist outwards, stretching the inner muscles of the forearm.

Start with simple exercises and enrich them as you learn about the meridians and feel your body: what it needs to become more flexible or more toned. The position should be held for about 8 breaths, but even longer if there is a feeling of discomfort or pain that gradually decreases.

Adding isometric stretching makes this exercise more complete: I stretch the muscle fascia; I inhale; I exhale and contract the outermost part of the muscle bundle (the part closest to the feet, hands, or the muscle segment that interests me); I inhale and try to stretch further. I should feel a slight improvement in flexibility after just 4-5 repetitions.

In any case, the principles are always the same:

1)   Do not hold your breath while exercising

2)   Do not feel pain: when you reach the pain threshold, the muscle contracts to defend itself and becomes counterproductive. If, on the other hand, you stretch too far beyond the pain threshold, you can damage the tendon, which then loses tone

3)   If you start to shake due to too much tension, loosen up, take a few breaths, and then return to the exercise, pulling a little less

4)   Keep your torso upright and not hunched over.

5)   Understand whether the discomfort brings relief (the Qi flows better) or whether it only causes discomfort, pain, or puts tension on a joint without keeping it aligned.

6)   Hold the position for at least 8 breaths.

8. QIGONG: BREATHING AND ENERGY

8.1 Introduction to Qigong

Qigong (also written as Qi Gong, Chi Kung, or Daoyin) is, in a nutshell, Chinese traditional health exercises. Its roots lie in shamanic practices, predating any written codification of meridians, points, Yin and Yang, and all the theoretical elements we have discussed so far. Dances or movements born and transmitted from the bodily experience of people who had a different attitude and perception of their own bodies. They used their bodies all day long to live: hunting, farming, building, producing artifacts... They were therefore subject to much more physical, mental, and environmental stress, so in moments of "refreshment," in addition to rest, they devoted themselves to movements and activities, possibly collective, to "stretch their muscles and strengthen their tendons, stretch the arch (of the head), and spread Qi throughout the body (through breathing)."

There was therefore an approach to exercise and movement that was not for work purposes but had nothing to do with the recreational or aesthetic - or even professional - aspects that it has taken on today.

Over time, Chinese medicine has become part of the practice of Qigong (who can say how much Qigong itself has influenced acupuncture, perhaps suggesting the existence of certain points that are particularly effective), and the practice itself has become one of the five pillars of Chinese medicine (along with acupuncture, massage, dietetics, and herbal medicine).

As mentioned earlier, Qigong is the only practice where the individual is responsible for themselves: they must strive to do themselves good, they must be constant, disciplined, and do it with attention and care because they are both the input and output of what they do: while other disciplines depend on external input, Qigong is an input that we ourselves create to obtain the output of well-being, healing, and health in general.

The term Qigong can take on different meanings: working with Qi, but also making Qi work. Qi is generically defined as "energy," the counterpart of Prana, Pneuma. Some define it as "breath," but this would be too narrow a definition with an exclusively materialistic connotation. Instead, Qi affects everything, both material and immaterial. Gong, on the other hand, is the part that characterizes the practice because it is not just work or practice, but a practice done with precision, dedication, attention, and presence. Therefore, when practicing Qigong, it is important t te attention to posture, the correct execution of movements, the fact that joints must be flexible but not loose, calm breathing, and a mind that is attentive and present to what is being done and does not wander to thoughts that distract it elsewhere. There must be no effort or pain, because this would block the flow of Qi and make the mind uncomfortable with the practice, seeing it as a form of stress. Each teacher will then provide the information necessary for a profitable and well-done practice, depending on the style practiced.

We talk about different styles because Qigong, like Kung Fu—its martial offspring—developed everywhere in China, characterized by numerous schools that differ from one another. It is said that there are 600. Perhaps the number is exaggerated, but if you consider that Ba Duan Jing (eight pieces of brocade), which is a sequence of eight movements, has many versions depending on whether it was developed by schools in the north or south, by a more martial school, in a colder region... you can search the internet and find at least seven or eight different versions, you will understand that as a discipline it can reach an incredible level of variety.

At a 'macro' level, Qigong can be classified as: Qigong for health (to maintain health or to heal certain pathologies/dysfunctions), martial Qigong (preparatory for martial arts), ' ' Qigong (in quotation marks because it would actually be more correct to define it as support for spiritual practices), which in turn can be divided into Taoist, Confucian, and Buddhist. In this discussion, we will only focus on Qigong for health or medical Qigong.

8.2. Medical Qigong

Medical Qigong is divided into two parts: internal and external. Internal Qi is developed through the individual practice of Qigong exercises. When those who practice Qigong become sufficiently skilled, they can use external Qi (waiQi in Chinese) to "transmit" Qi for the purpose of healing other people. This therapy has limited large-scale application, as there are few masters skilled in Qigong. However, we will focus on internal Qi, as almost anyone can learn Qigong exercises to maintain health and promote self-healing.

In the early 1980s, scientists in China began to study the numerous therapeutic benefits claimed by Qigong. Since then, research on hundreds of medical applications of Qigong has been reported in Chinese medical literature. A large amount of material has also been published in English following an increase in international conferences. Since 1986, 837 abstracts have been published, more than half of them in English. The English abstracts have been entered into a database to enable searches using keywords and to expand bibliographies.

Below are specific studies and evidence designed to identify and measure the beneficial effects of Qigong.

Several examples of medical applications of Qigong and Qi emitted on humans, animals, and plants have been examined. Clinical and experimental evidence shows that the practice of

Qigong and external Qi affect various functions and organs of the body. Some of the functions and organs affected by Qigong, and the related measurement techniques, include the brain (electroencephalogram [EEG] and magnetometry), blood flow (thermography, sphygmography, and roentencephalography), cardiac functions (blood pressure, electrocardiogram, and ultrasonic cardiogram), kidneys (urine albumin rate), biophysics (enzyme activity, immune function, sex hormone levels), visual acuity, and tumor size in mice.

Below, we will examine some experimental and clinical research studies to illustrate the relevance of research on the medical applications of Qigong. Studies containing scientific information related to medical conditions have been selected.

Therapeutic balance of meridians and body functions

The effects of Qigong practice on the therapeutic rebalancing of the meridian system and body functions can be monitored with Voll's electroacupuncture (EAV). In EAV, the electrical conductance of the skin at individual acupuncture points is measured using low voltage and low current. The diagnosis depends on the relative electrical conductance and its dependence on time. An important diagnostic criterion for organ degeneration is a "drop in the indicator" that can occur during measurement, when the conductance reaches an apparent maximum value but then decreases before stabilizing.

146

The measurements were taken by the same operator and with the same instruments on 24 acupuncture points at the end of the meridians of the subjects' fingers and toes. The subjects were asked to perform a Qigong exercise of their choice, for example, sitting or standing meditation, or moving Qigong. Two series of EAV measurements were taken before and after the healthy subjects practiced Qigong. In the first series, four subjects were examined with EAV before and after practicing Qigong for 10 to 15 minutes. For the four subjects, Qigong practice decreased the average EAV values measured by 19% to 31% (P<.004, note 2). In essence, Qigong eliminated the decline in the indicator. In the second series, each of the seven subjects was examined with EAV in three stages using a blind protocol, so that the operator did not know whether a subject had practiced Qigong before the second or third examination. Qigong practice decreased the average EAV values measured from 17% to 35% for four subjects ( ) and increased them from 4% to 15% in three subjects. Again, the decline in the indicator was reduced.

These preliminary results show that Qigong can produce significant changes in the therapeutic balance of meridians and organ systems, which is the goal of TCM.

Hypertension

In China, some groups have studied the effects of Qigong on hypertension. Research on the short- and long-term effects of

Qigong practice on patients with hypertension was conducted at the Institute of Hypertension in Shanghai by Wang et al. Their research serves as a model for the effects of Qigong on many bodily functions. For these studies, patients practiced "Yan Jing Shen Gong" for 30 minutes twice a day. This Qigong exercise, which is believed to be particularly effective for therapeutic purposes and for delaying aging, consists of a combination of seated meditation and gentle physical movements that increase calmness of mind, relaxation of the body, and regular breathing.

Heart attack and mortality

In 1991, researchers presented a 20-year controlled study on the anti-aging effects of Qigong on 204 patients with hypertension. Recently, researchers conducted a 30-year follow-up study on 242 patients with hypertension who had been randomly divided into a Qigong group (n=122) and a control group (n=120). All patients received drug therapy to control blood pressure, but only the experimental group practiced Qigong for 30 minutes twice a day. The results show that the total mortality rate was 25.41% in the Qigong group and 40.8% in the control group (P<.001). The incidence of heart attack was 20.5% and 40.7% (P<.01), respectively, and the expected mortality rate following the attack was 15.6% and 32.5%, respectively.

The researchers also reported that after a period of 20 years, the blood pressure of the Qigong group had stabilized, while that of the control group had increased. It should be noted that during this period, the dosage of medication for the Qigong group could be reduced and for 30% of patients it could be eliminated. On the contrary, for the control group it was necessary to increase the dosage of medication.

Cardiac function and microcirculation

Older patients with hypertension usually have a deficiency of heart energy, which often causes functional weakening of the left ventricle and microcirculation disorders. In a study of 120 male subjects aged between 55 and 75, researchers evaluated the effects of Qigong using ultrasonic cardiography and microcirculation indices ( ). The subjects were divided into three groups: 46 subjects with hypertension and Heart energy deficiency, 34 without Heart energy deficiency, and 40 with normal blood pressure. Patients with blood pressure above 160/95 mmHg were included after adjusting their blood pressure with antihypertensive drugs for 4 weeks.

The results showed that subjects with heart energy deficiency experienced some improvements: increases in cardiac power, ejection fraction, diastolic mitral valve closure velocity, and mean fiber circumference decrease velocity, while total peripheral resistance decreased (P<.05-.01). No significant changes occurred in the group without cardiac energy deficiency.

Multiple quantitative assessment of microcirculation disorders at the lateral edge of the nail was performed on the three groups by examining 10 indices of abnormal conditions: micrangium (terminal microcapillary) configuration, micrangium tension, blood flow conditions, blood flow slowing, thinner afferent branch, efferent and afferent branch ratio, blood color, hemorrhage, and petechiae. At the beginning of the study, the incidence of microcirculation obstruction was 73.9%, 26.5%, and 17.5% for the three groups, respectively. After practicing Qigong for 1 year, the group with cardiac energy deficiency showed a significant decrease in microcirculation obstruction at the nail margin from 73.9% to 39.3% (P<.05). No significant changes were observed in the group without cardiac energy deficiency. The researchers emphasized that Qigong practice should be chosen taking into account the condition of the patients.

Sex hormone levels

One of the consequences of aging is that sex hormone levels change in unfavorable directions. For example, the level of the female hormone (estrogen) tends to increase in men and decrease in women. Studies indicate that this trend can be reversed with Qigong practice.

In a study on the effects of Qigong practice on plasma sex hormone levels in men and women with hypertension, sex hormone levels were measured before and after 1 year of Qigong practice. The 70 male patients with essential hypertension (aged 40 to 69 years; disease grade II) were divided into two groups. In the Qigong group (n=42), the estradiol level decreased from 70 to 47.7 pg/mL, a decrease of 32% (P<.01), while no significant changes were found in the control group (n=20). In both groups, the testosterone level decreased by 7%. The estradiol value for the Qigong group (47.7 pg/mL) was close to that of a healthy man (42.2±5.8 pg/mL) of the same age but without hypertension or cardiovascular, pulmonary, renal, hepatic, or endocrine diseases (P<.05). For women (aged 51 to 67 years; number of subjects unavailable), the aging process was associated with ovarian insufficiency manifested by decreased estradiol levels and increased testosterone levels. Qigong produced an increase in estradiol from 40.9±3.5 to 51.6±3.5 pg/mL, a value almost equal to that of normal menopause in control subjects without hypertension or cardiovascular, pulmonary, hepatic, or endocrine diseases. Testosterone levels also increased with Qigong from 25.5 ± 2.3 to 37.2 ± 2.2 ng/dL.

In an additional study, 24-hour urinary estradiol levels were measured in 30 men aged 50 to 69 years. Practicing Qigong for 1 year resulted in a 31% decrease in estradiol and a 54% decrease in the estradiol-to-testosterone ratio. These changes were accompanied by improvements in symptoms such as pain, dizziness, insomnia, hair loss, impotence, and incontinence

151

associated with kidney deficiency hypertension (according to a TCM diagnosis). With Qigong, the average score for these symptoms decreased from 5.5 ± 2.3 to 2.8 ± 1.3 (P < .001).

Ye and colleagues reported similar significant changes in plasma estradiol levels in 77 men and women who had practiced Qigong for 2 months, compared with 27 control subjects , for whom no significant change in testosterone levels was observed.

Bone density

With aging, bone density decreases, especially in women. As a result, bones become more fragile and prone to fractures. It was found that bone density had increased in male subjects who had been practicing Qigong for 1 year. In 18 subjects aged between 50 and 59, bone density had increased from 0.627 ± 0.040 to 0.696 ± 0.069 g/cm3. In 12 subjects aged 60 to 69, bone density had increased slightly less: from 0.621 ± 0.039 to 0.672 ± 0.083 g/cm3. For both age groups, bone density increased to values exceeding those of a normal man of the same age, by 0.695 ± 0.096 and 0.657 ± 0.102 g/cm3, respectively.

It seems likely that this Qigong therapy can also restore bone density in women, especially those in menopause. In this case, hormone replacement therapy and its side effects could be reduced.

Chemical changes in the blood of patients with hypertension

Further studies conducted by Xu and colleagues on the effects of Qigong practice on blood chemistry in subjects with hypertension showed improvements in plasma fibrinolysin coagulation indices, blood visco , erythrocyte deformation index, plasma plasminogen activator level, plasminogen activator inhibitor, factor VIII antigen, and antithrombin III. In another study, they reported that Qigong practice had significantly and beneficially altered the activity of two cyclic messenger nucleotides (cyclic adenosine monophosphate and cyclic guanosine monophosphate).

Cancer

In the Qigong Database, the terms cancer, carcinoma, or tumor appear in the titles of 62 abstracts. Feng's pioneering research showed that the Qi emitted by Qigong masters produced marked changes in cancer cell cultures in mice. Some studies have reported the effects of emitted Qi on tumors in animals. For example, it has been reported that emitted Qi inhibits the growth of malignant tumors implanted in mice but does not destroy the tumors. Encouraged by the results obtained in animals, researchers have conducted clinical studies on the effects of Qigong on human subjects with cancer. Detailed results are not available in English for any of these clinical studies.

Some results are available from a clinical study on Qigong as a therapeutic aid for patients with advanced cancer. In this study, patients with a medical diagnosis of malignant cancer were divided into a group of 97 patients who practiced Qigong and a control group of 30 patients. All subjects were taking medication, and the study group practiced Qigong for more than 2 hours a day for a period of 3 to 6 months. Both groups experienced improvements, but the study group showed improvements in strength, appetite, absence of diarrhea, and weight gain (3 kg) that were four to nine times greater than the control group. The phagocytic rate, which is a measure of immune function, increased in the Qigong group and decreased in the control group.

Senility

To study the mechanism by which physical fitness is maintained through Qigong, a controlled study was conducted on 100 subjects, classified as either presenile or with brain function deficits due to senility. The subjects were divided into two groups of 50 people; each group had an average age of 62.7 years and a similar distribution by age and gender. The Qigong group practiced a combination of static and moving Qigong. The control group exercised by walking, brisk walking, or slow running. Based on the TCM method of classifying vital energy, more than 80% of the patients in each group were classified as deficient in vital function and vital essence of the Kidney. The criteria for evaluating the outcome were based on the measurement of clinical signs and symptoms including: brain function, sexual function, serum lipid levels, and endocrine gland function.

154

After 6 months, 8 of the 14 main clinical signs and symptoms had improved by more than 80% in the Qigong group, while in the control group none of the symptoms had improved by more than 45%.

Mind-body regulation

The main function of Qigong is to regulate the mind, particularly brain functions and related bodily reactions. One of the principles of Qigong is that the mind guides Qi, and Qi guides blood. This somewhat mysterious statement can be interpreted to mean that intention (the mind) can direct Qi within the body. This mechanism is probably similar to the role of willpower in self-regulation through biofeedback.

Brain waves

Research has focused primarily on the effects of Qigong on brain waves measured by electroencephalogram (EEG). During meditation, whether standing or sitting, alpha brain waves prevail over beta waves and spread to the frontal areas of the brain.

Kawano and Wang found differences in the electroencephalograms of Zen Buddhist monks and Qigong masters. During almost all types of Qigong practice, the frequency of alpha waves increased from 0.6 to 1.0 Hz. During deep Zen meditation, the frequency decreased from -1.0 to -1.5 Hz, and theta waves sometimes appeared. In addition, frontal and occipital alpha waves tended to synchronize with a different phase depending on the type of meditation. This phase difference became smaller with Qigong meditation (i.e., synchronization was better) and larger with Zen meditation. According to Kawano and Wang, these differences in brain function suggest that internal Qigong is a semi-unconscious process involving a certain amount of awareness and activity, while Zen meditation is a neutral process that frees the meditator from all worries. Perhaps because of this difference, Qigong is considered a healthy art, while Zen generally is not.

As mentioned earlier, a Qigong master can emit Qi to heal a patient. The interaction between Qigong masters and subjects was simultaneously evaluated using EEG, polygraph tests, biochemical blood tests, and psychological tests. The analyzed EEGs showed that the type of brain waves and their location were synchronized in the brains of the Qigong masters and the subjects. Such synchronism may be required for healing through emitted Qi.

Machi compared the EEG results with simultaneous measurements of physiological changes in the Qigong masters. He found that while the Qigong master emitted Qi, alpha-1 waves showed extremely high potential in the right frontal lobe and increased blood pressure, heart rate, and skin surface temperature. He also discovered infrared emission with a 1Hz modulation signal coming from the Laogong point (an important acupuncture point on the palm of the hand).

Blood flow to the brain

Roentgenencephalography has shown that practicing Qigong increases blood flow to the brain. In 158 subjects with cerebral arteriosclerosis who had practiced Qigong for 1 to 6 months, improvements were noted in symptoms such as memory, dizziness, insomnia, tinnitus,

Rapid and extensive changes in altitude

Studies have been conducted to determine whether Qigong practice can protect pilots from altitude stress when they move quickly from low altitudes to the mountainous areas of Tibet.

Cardiac function. Before arriving in the Tibetan mountain areas, 66 young men were divided into two groups: a group of 32 subjects who had practiced Qigong Qiyuan for 4 weeks and a control group who had trained while listening to music. The two groups were suddenly taken from a lower altitude to the mountain areas. Before and after the ascent, measurements were taken of altitude sickness symptoms and physiological changes. The Qigong group suffered less from altitude stress than the control group, as measured by blood pressure, heart rate, oxygen consumption, microcirculation at the tip of the tongue and nail margin, and temperature at the Laogong (P8) point of the left hand (P<.01). Some researchers have also reported the beneficial effects of Qigong on cardiovascular disorders.

Microcirculation disorders. In a study on microcirculation, 40 military pilots were randomly divided into two groups: a group of 22 subjects who had practiced Qigong Qiyuan for 8 weeks, and a control group of 18 who had practiced physical exercises before arriving in the mountainous areas of Tibet. Microcirculation was measured at the tip of the tongue and the nail margin, and temperature was measured at the Laogong point on the palm of the left hand. When a subject was at the highest altitude, blood pressure and microcirculation at the tip of the tongue and nail margin were abnormal in both groups. However, the abnormalities were statistically smaller in the study group than in the control group (P<.01). The temperature of Laogong remained constant in the study group and decreased in the control group (P<.05).

Lung function. In a study of lung function, 120 young people were divided into three groups of 40 subjects each. Group 1 had practiced Qigong Qiyuan for 4 weeks before arriving at higher altitudes; group 2, the control group, had trained for 4 weeks listening to music on the radio before arriving at higher altitudes; group 3 consisted of subjects who lived permanently at high altitudes. The results showed that the integral value of acute mountain sickness symptoms was lower in the Qigong group than

158

in the control group (P<.05-.01). The pulmonary ventilation of the Qigong group was significantly improved compared to that of the control group (P<.05-.01), and was almost equal to that of the resident group.

Combination of Qigong and medication versus medication alone

There is ample evidence in the literature that a therapy combining self-practiced Qigong and medication is superior to drug therapy alone. This conclusion is reported in many studies on hypertension and in the treatment of cancer patients. The advantages of a combination of Qigong and medication over medication alone have already been described.

The mechanism of this evident synergy is unknown, but it undoubtedly involves the fundamental mechanism of Qigong. Qigong is believed to relax the body, promote the flow of Qi (energy), blood, oxygen, and nutrients to all cells in the body, and rid the cells of waste products. Improvements in Qi flow and microcirculation nourish diseased or stressed tissues. We can hypothesize that Qigong also promotes the absorption of drugs by tissues and cells through improved microcirculation.

8.3 Qigong exercises

In the previous chapter, we already covered the essential aspects of movement and breathing, which are the pillars of good and correct Qigong practice (and any sports discipline). Posture is another pillar that requires maximum attention and can be summarized in the following key points:

1)   The feet are normally parallel and the weight is mainly carried on the 'hard' part of the foot, i.e. the bone that runs from the heel, along the outside, to the forefoot. There are positions where the feet are together, shoulder-width apart (let's say this is the most common position), or wider than shoulder-width apart.

2)   The knees are 'unlocked', i.e. they are not straight but slightly bent without straining the quadriceps.

3)   The pelvis is free to move, the groin area must be relaxed (without tension or contraction), and the coccyx must be positioned at an angle halfway between "tail between the legs" – where I rotate the pelvis until the lumbar curve is flattened – and "tail out" – where I reverse the rotation and try to maximize the lumbar curve.

4)   The shoulders are relaxed and the shoulder blades are well positioned and connected to the rib cage.

5)   The head is suspended in the sky: the top of the head points towards the sky and the chin is brought slightly back and towards the sternum in order to minimize the cervical curve.

6)   I should not feel any muscle tension, fatigue, or joint stiffness; my breathing is deep and reaches below my navel. Each limb should take on the appearance of an arch, i.e., it should have

160

curves (albeit slight) and should not have any sharp edges or be a straight line.

7)   The Baihui point (top of the head) should be aligned with the center of the perineum (Huiyin) and with the center of the square formed by the feet. This axis connecting the earth with the sky should be as close as possible to the spine.

8)   The mind is calm and relaxed and focused on the body and the sensations it sends us when we move or even just stand in a posture. I do not think about what I have to do next, what happened yesterday, or the work I will have to do in the coming days, because those activities will have their moment of maximum attention: when practicing Qigong, you practice Qigong; when eating pizza, you eat pizza; when writing an email, you write an email. we must learn to tame our mind, and breathing is the first h l tool that helps us in this incredible, incredibly complicated process.

Exercise 1)

From the basic posture, which involves keeping your feet perpendicular to each other (which will bring your feet to shoulder width), relax your arms along your sides and support your head with the entire structure that starts at your heels, rises along your spine, and reaches your neck. The head is like a capital on the spine; there is no tension, but there is a feeling of upward thrust. Imagine that a sap rises from the soles of your feet, travels up your legs, crosses your pelvis, rises along your spine, reaches your shoulders, and then descends along your arms and 'drips' from your hands. I repeat this sap rise a few times until I feel my legs, trunk, and arms become 'fuller' and more energetic. At that point, my sap has filled my body and can rise up my neck, fill my skull, and then flow out from the Baihui point and down my body, enveloping it as if it were warm ambrosia that warms, illuminates, and nourishes my skin. This exercise requires no effort, only the ability to give yourself time to be, breathe deeply, and move the Qi along the earth/sky axis with visualization.

Benefits: harmonizes Qi, regulates blood pressure, slows the heart rate, helps to spread Qi throughout the body, releasing tension and spreading warmth throughout the body.

Exercise 2)

From the position in exercise 1, inhale while standing on your tiptoes for a moment, raise your shoulders and rotate them backward, arch your back and lift your chest (do not collapse your lower back), and look up. Then, as you exhale, bend forward, rolling your spine (starting from the head, chest, back, and lower back) and massage the outer side of your legs with your hands as you descend. Once you have finished exhaling, reach your hands towards your feet, move onto the inner side of your legs, bend your knees slightly to support the rise and, as you inhale, rise up, unrolling your spine (lower back, back, chest, head) and finish the inhalation by going back onto your toes and rotating your shoulders. Perform 9 cycles (corresponding to 9 complete breaths). Do this slowly and carefully, keeping your hands on your body, so that when you rise, they do not come away from your body and your elbows do not lift.

Benefits: stimulates and stretches the entire posterior chain (urinary bladder and Du Mai meridians) and stimulates the stomach meridian ( ) located on the front of the body, stimulates the KI1 point, pushes Qi along the gallbladder meridians and the Yin meridians of the legs.

Exercise 3)

Horse stance (feet wider than shoulder width apart, lower yourself toward the ground as if to sit down: find the ideal height based on the effort required for a position that is too low—do not go below 90 degrees at the knee joint—and without straining the lower back). With your hands, draw circles perpendicular to your torso, alternating the movement of your hands: as one hand rises, touching your sternum, then moves forward and descends, the other hand descends, moves towards your navel and rises along the center line, touching your sternum. Breathe freely and repeat 20 circles with each hand. The torso is not rotated, it always remains facing forward. After completing the 20 circles, the hands, starting from the iliac crests, make an alternating "forward/backward" movement: one advances from the iliac crest, slides over the abdomen to the navel and from there detaches from the body and stretches forward, without fully extending the elbow. Meanwhile, the other hand is brought slightly back, remaining on the side, pushing the elbow back as far as possible but without excessive strain that could cause contractures or strains. The shoulders rotate very widely, in a r manner, causing an energetic twisting of the torso. Repeat 20 times on each side. Once this movement is complete, spread your arms out to the sides with your elbows bent and your palms facing upwards as if you were carrying two large trays. Bend your knees slightly so that you are 10-15 cm higher than the horse stance. From this position, rotate your arms forward, keeping your elbows bent, as if you were going to tip the trays onto the floor. turn your palms downwards and bend your knees, returning to the horse stance; then rotate your arms, bringing your palms forward and then back up again (as if holding the trays), rising 10-15 cm from the horse stance, but without fully extending your legs. Repeat the double movement of rising and lowering 20 times. Finally, draw large circles with your arms, bringing your hands down, crossing your arms, your right hand rising on the left side and your left hand rising on the right side. Raise your arms, bringing your hands above your head (up to this point, your palms are facing your body), rotate your palms outward, and each hand descends sideways on its respective side. The legs follow the movement of the arms, bending when the hands go down and cross, then stretching out when the arms rise. Compared to the previous movement, the legs have a freer, less controlled movement and should be lighter after the previous 3 sets , which may have been tiring. The movement is repeated 20 times.

Benefits: Strengthens the legs, involving the stomach and kidney meridians. Controls the Ming Men area, which is strengthened. Balances the water-fire relationship: in the first two movements, attention is focused on the little finger and middle finger (fire). The second movement also works on the belt vessel, balancing the upper and lower body. In the last two movements, it is important to focus on the mobility of the shoulder blades, which has beneficial effects on the heart. The twisting movement of the spine in the second movement is beneficial for the immune system (cleansing of the marrow).

Exercise 4)

Take a step forward with your left foot while pointing your right foot outwards (the toes are therefore pointing left and right). Remain slightly seated on your knees, place your hands on your hips and then, imagining you are kneading a large ball, make circles in an anti-clockwise direction: the movement starts from the feet, rotate the pelvis in an anti-clockwise direction and follow with the torso, then the trunk, shoulders and finally the hands, as if there were resistance in the 'ball' being kneaded. The hands draw a quarter circle, positioning themselves in front, and then return to the hips. Continue the counterclockwise movement of the pelvis, torso, nd trunk, bring the hands back to the right, and start again. Make 9 counterclockwise circles starting from the right, then reverse the position of the feet and make 9 clockwise circles from the left.

Benefits: hip mobility, frees the belt vessel by balancing the upper and lower body, charges and concentrates energy in the palms of the hands (useful for massage therapists), preparatory exercise for many Taijiquan applications.

Exercise 5)

Raise your hands forward with your arms extended (press your index finger into the corner of your nail with your thumb), bring your left foot behind and to the right of your right foot (crossing your legs), shift your weight onto both feet and squat down while bringing your hands close to your chest. Push your hands forward and stand up again, keeping your legs crossed. Squat down again, bring your hands close to your chest, then extend them to the right at an angle of about 45 degrees and stand up. Squat down a

166

third time and again bring your hands close to your chest, then extend them to the right at an angle of about 90 degrees. From this low position, bring your left hand to your left side (your arms are now stretched out at your sides), then bring your hands forward with your arms stretched out, lift yourself up, and return your feet to the starting position. Repeat the same movement symmetrically on the other side, then repeat it again on both sides.

Benefits: strengthens the legs and tendons, stimulates the lungs (the position of the fingers is held with moderate pressure and stimulates the lung and large intestine points), the twist stimulates the belt vessel, thus balancing the upper and lower body, and deepens the breath because the movement is done very slowly: inhale before squatting and while standing up, exhale while squatting.

Exercise 6)

Lift your left foot, bringing your left thigh to 90 degrees and bending your knee, swing your hands backward to make a sideways circle and, gaining speed in the fall, slap the ST36 point with your left hand and the SP9 point with your right hand on the bent leg. Then bring your left foot to the ground and lift your right leg, slapping the same points ST36 and SP9. Do this 4 times on each side and then do the same movement but hit the points with your hands closed in a fist - not clenched but empty: you can look inside. $ times on each side.

Benefits: improves balance and stimulates the rectus femoris muscles, and therefore the entire stomach meridian muscle line; works on the earth points of the earth (stomach and spleen), thus supporting and strengthening both organs, improving moisture transformation and strengthening the legs.

8.4. Specific exercises for earth and metal

Earth controls muscle structure and flesh, while metal controls the skin, but in this system, attention is focused on the functions of the lungs and large intestine. Therefore, EARTH as structure will involve muscle-type exercises, while METAL is closely linked to earth, not only because in the 'family' relationship it is the child of earth, but also because according to the nomenclature of Chinese meridians, there are not 12 but 6, divided as follows:

-       Taiyin: Lung/Spleen

-       Shaoyin: Heart / Kidneys

-       Jueyin: Liver / Pericardium

-       Yang Ming: Stomach / Large intestine

-       Tai Yang: Bladder / Small Intestine

-       Shaoyang: Gallbladder / Triple heater.

It is immediately apparent that the earth and metal meridians belong to the same energy level. Water and fire are also closely connected (Shaoyin and Taiyang). However, since it is always good to strengthen the earth in any situation (whether to maintain, improve, or recover from an illness or surgery), and since this is not the place to discuss Qigong in depth, you can learn more at with a good teacher, possibly assisted by a good manual (and not vice versa).

The following series is moderately intense from a muscular point of view and includes positions on the ground and standing up.

Earth has the function of transforming, metal of assimilating and protecting.

Position 1)

Sitting cross-legged, pinch the big toe and the first toe of the foot respectively at the well points of the SP and ST meridians using the thumb and index finger of the hand, specifically with the nail angle of the thumb (LU well point) and index finger (LI well point). In practice, the respective well points of the Yang Ming and Tai Yin meridians are brought into contact. Inhale and press with increasing intensity until you reach the end of the inhalation. Release the pressure and hold your breath for a moment. Then exhale and press again as before with increasing intensity until the end of the exhalation, at which point you release the pressure and hold your breath again for a moment. Do this for 10 complete breaths. It may be helpful to think of two words, one for the inhalation phase and one for the exhalation phase (inhale/exhale, slow/deep, gather/let go...).

170

Position 2)

Bring one knee up to your chest while keeping the other leg extended. Remain seated on your sitting bones and never rest your feet during the exercise. The foot of the extended leg is in a hammer position while the foot of the bent leg is extended. With the hand on the side of the bent leg, press the thenar eminence, pressing the ST36 area, and with the index and middle fingers, press the SP9 area. Then alternate legs and grasp the knee with the other hand. Inhale and extend one leg, exhale and extend the other leg. Repeat 10 times on each side.

Position 3)

Extend your legs, place your hands on the ground next to your pelvis with your fingers pointing forward. Resting on your heels, lift your pelvis, trying to form an inclined plane with your body from your heels to your shoulders. Hold the raised position for 4 breaths and then lower yourself. Repeat, rotating your hands 90 degrees: now your fingers are pointing outwards. Finally, repeat a third time, rotating your hands another 90 degrees: your fingers are pointing backward. In this position, it is important to feel your chest opening (you can space your hands slightly apart as this is the most strenuous position).

Position 4)

Turn into position without (sitting on your heels with your legs bent). Extend your arms and raise your hands (which are not joined) forward with your fingers pointing downwards (so as to extend the LI meridian well). When your hands reach shoulder height, make a pistol grip with your hands (thumb and index finger extended and other fingers closed) and rotate your palms upward. Then bring your hands outwards, still at shoulder height. Then open your hands and close them into fists starting with your little fingers, bend your wrists and elbows, and bring your hands close to your shoulders, creating a slight isometric resistance (as if elastic bands were making it difficult to bring them together). Once your hands are at your shoulders, open them and slide the backs of your hands along your chest, stretching your hands backward with a slight twist and extending only your index finger (again, maximum extension of the LI meridian): be careful not to close your shoulders forward, but keep your chest open. Then move into the seated camel position, resting your palms on the balls of your feet. Repeat twice and vary the position when you make the pistol fingers: bend your head once to the right and once to the left and hold for the entire next phase.

Position 5)

Get on all fours and start with 3 "cow-cat" movements: inhale and arch your back, bringing your chin up; exhale and hunch your back, bringing your chin towards your sternum. With your hands shoulder-width apart, rest on your toes and do the plank, keeping your abs and glutes tight. Your chin should be facing your sternum and your gaze should be towards your feet below. Hold the position for 5 breaths. Then move into a triangle position, slightly widening your feet for greater stability. Keep your head tucked in between your shoulders and your buttocks as high as possible. Arms and legs extended. Hold the position for 5 breaths. Next, bend your arms and stay in a low platform position: your body is raised a few centimeters off the ground and your abs are tense. Hold the position for as long as you can, up to 5 breaths. Finally, move into the cobra position: extend your arms, trying to keep your pelvis as close to the ground as possible; your feet are resting on the backs of your heels (so as to stretch the ST meridian at the ankles) and your chin is pointing upwards. Hold the position for 5 full breaths. Repeat the sequence 3 times and each time you complete a cycle, repeat the "cow-cat" movements 5 times.

Position 6)

Standing. Bring your palms together and raise your arms, keeping the LI meridian extended (fingertips pointing downwards), and bring your hands above your head, arms fully extended. Inhale deeply and as you exhale, bring your hands slightly behind your shoulders. Hold the position for a few seconds (your shoulders should not be raised) and then, with your hands still together, bend your arms and bring your hands together at your chest. Press your hands firmly against each other and, as you take three breaths, increase the pressure of your hands as you exhale. Then inhale deeply, hold your breath for a moment, contracting all your muscles and the root (perineum), and then exhale explosively, thrusting your hands forward as if throwing a spear. Keeping them in contact on the edge of the hand, turn the palms of the hands upwards, then rotate the hands towards the chest, joining the backs of the hands, and perform 3 complete rotations, ensuring that the shoulders also rotate widely to accompany the movement. After the third rotation, bring your hands, joined only at the thenar eminence, towards the dantian. Repeat the sequence 3 times.

Position 7)

Standing. Elbows raised to shoulder height and to the sides, fingertips touching. Open your arms outwards (inhaling) and when your arms are stretched out, rotate your palms upwards (pinky finger up and index finger down) and close them in the starting position (exhaling). 10 breathing cycles. Extend the HT and SI meridians when opening and the LI and LU meridians when closing, then move your wrists.

Position 8)

Walking. Take a half-moon step and lower yourself into a horse stance. If the right foot is forward, bring the right hand (thenar eminence) to the left groin to press the ST30 area. In this way, the body is rotated 90 degrees to the left relative to the direction of walking. The left arm, with the left hand resting on the left hip, extends sideways and draws a semicircle clockwise, and with the hand (palm down) makes a gathering movement. Moving forward, rotate the pelvis and the entire torso forward, then return to the starting position and bring the left hand to the left hip. At this point, perform a block/strike with the left hand, with the palm and fingers facing outward. The right hand slides from the left groin area to the right hip and the left leg (back leg) is extended. The torso is facing forward. Now step forward with your left leg and repeat the sequence on the other side. Repeat 3 times on each side. Important te the intention of gathering and then pushing the Qi. The hand on ST30 should sink slightly. If the area is too tense, you need to tilt your pelvis backward.

Position 9)

Self-massage. Bring your right hand under your left armpit and your left hand under your right armpit. Your right arm is lower. Slide your hands towards the opposite side until they reach the inguinal fossa (right on the right and left on the left, the left hand passes over the navel and the right hand under the navel) and then slide along the ST meridian with the thenar eminence, pressing vigorously. Pinch the ankles for a moment and then move up, pressing with the thenar eminence on the SP meridian. Center the hands on the midline, with the right hand remaining higher and resting on the center of the sternum with the thenar eminence, while the left hand remains resting below the navel. Then, breathing slowly, lower the right hand with light pressure until it reaches above the left hand.

As you descend, your back curls up, and as you ascend, it uncurls, bending in the following order: head, cervical, dorsal, and lumbar, and then stretching in the following order: lumbar, dorsal, cervical, and head.

Position 10)

Repeat position 1 for at least 10 complete breaths.

176

9. OUR BODY GIVES US INFORMATION

9.1. Listening to and reading our bodies – a practical analysis

As mentioned in the introduction, the goal we should set ourselves is to keep illness at bay or be able to respond effectively to illness and eliminate it quickly and permanently. You have probably come across people who explain that illness is a sign, a message that we must interpret. To correct certain habits or certain directions in our lives. Illness does not want to hurt us but wants us to be better, and illness arises when we try to solve a problem (which we are probably not even aware of because it is so deep-seated). Unfortunately, this is indeed the case, but since the argument is very uncertain and the investigation involves study, time, effort, and research, modern medicine has not even wasted time labeling these theories. They do not exist. Period. Then we cannot explain why champions of Ronaldo's caliber collapse emotionally during the most important final of their careers, even though they are physically at their peak. Didn't he have a mental coach? If the answer is "no," then perhaps he needed one. If the answer is "yes," then perhaps he was unaware of certain energetic elements of his client that went beyond physical health and goal visualization. And how many times have you (or someone you know) had an injury just before an important decision? And on which side of the body? Ignoring the fact that I am more likely to sprain my ankle than suffer whiplash means not wanting to interpret these messages. They are not necessarily esoteric, perhaps they are simply caused by poor posture, a body posture that stresses the joints. But in order to intervene, we must start from the principle: "Know thyself," and only we are responsible for this, no one else.

We will discuss certain anatomical parts, identifying their psychosomatic and energetic significance. In this way, we will try to provide keys to understanding that we can then apply to other parts of the body. The choice was made based on the frequency of disorders affecting these areas of our body.

The ankle.

The ankle is basically the link, the bridge between myself and the earth, the material world; all problems with this joint express a conflict with the earth and everything it represents, from femininity and the relationship with the mother to material things (money, work, security).

It symbolizes the projection of our ability to decide, to take responsibility for decisions and changes in our lives, to get involved.

The ankle: it allows us to express our ability to make decisions, to change our position in life. The ground symbolizes reality and the ankle gives us stability or mobility in relation to reality as we perceive it.

A sprain or twist almost always expresses a refusal to conform to a direction that is imposed on us: "WE ARE WALKING IN THE WRONG DIRECTION!!" "Did I want to cut ties with the authority of...?" "Do I have the impression that someone wants to 'control me or impose a path on me'?"

It symbolizes the final joint and represents the points of support and reference in our relationship with the world, in relation to others and ourselves.

The way we place our feet and therefore use our ankles is a faithful projection of the stability, rigidity, or flexibility of our positions and our conscious life criteria.

Ankle problems tell us about our relationship problems when we lack stability or flexibility. They indicate that we are going through a phase in which our positions, our life criteria, and the way we officially present ourselves to others no longer suit us, do not satisfy us, but we find it difficult to change them and move on.

The ankle also expresses our ability to jump, to take risks, to fly, so to speak, and not just keep our feet on the ground. All ankle injuries are like signals that perhaps we are running too fast, that perhaps we are not keeping our feet on the ground, that perhaps we should learn to do fewer things but do them well.

The ankle allows the foot to move, and problems in this joint can also indicate that we are on the wrong path; an accident (sprain or fracture) is an opportunity to stop and reflect.

As a result, the ankle also ends up stiffening in a completely unnatural way and, under stressful conditions, increased muscle tension increases the likelihood of sprains.

There are also people who develop a real tendency to this type of accident, not only because after the first truly traumatic sprain the ligaments become loose, but also because they find a predisposition in their emotional and physical states, the latter in terms of latent fatigue.

Some authors (Dahlke) see sprains as a kind of punishment for a mistake made, for a wrong committed to others; it is our superego that informs us of our mistake and punishes us in some way.

Therefore, we must take responsibility and acknowledge our mistakes.

A weak ankle, which will then lead to a sprain, always expresses a difficulty in bearing oneself, the weight of life, what we are doing; a clear signal: you have to hurt yourself in order to stop and reflect, perhaps the direction in your life is not quite right.

The Chinese view on this type of trauma is very clear; ice is never good because it somehow blocks blood circulation and therefore prolongs the period of pain and inflammation.

Ice appears to reduce inflammation, but in reality it blocks the blood that nourishes and actually reduces inflammation.

Therefore, strong massage with camphor oil and moxa on the painful areas are techniques that improve the situation more quickly.

Ice makes the inflamed area hard and difficult to treat.

IF THERE IS NO SWELLING, THE 'SPRAIN' IS MINOR

Four degrees of severity have been established for sprains, which doctors identify from zero to three, from least to most serious. In any case, the use of ice is the first form of intervention to be adopted.

In Chinese medicine, ice is used with caution for ankle sprains only on the first day to relieve pain, then massage can be started on the reflex zones: hands, head, feet, and then continued on the meridians involved, without ever treating the affected area (before and after the trauma). From the third or fourth day, you can also start massaging the affected area with a good warming oil and begin exercises to restore joint mobility and tendon strength. Of course, for major trauma, it is necessary to check that there are no injuries that require more invasive interventions and therapies, including surgery.

Finally, according to Chinese medicine, the ankle area is home to the Yuan points of the leg meridians, i.e., those points from which it is possible to draw the original energy of those energy lodges (not only the organs): bladder, gallbladder, stomach, spleen, pancreas, kidney, and liver. A mobile joint allows the Yuan energy of these lodges to be stimulated through exercises and movements. Is this important? Yes, both because being mobile on our legs and feet makes us freer to move around, and because giving energy and moving energy in all the energy lodges is necessary to avoid imbalances, both organic (blood circulation, for example) and energetic (liver Qi deficiency).

To conclude, the ankle is the pathway of water. The yuan points of the kidney, spleen, and liver meridians are located there. The Yin meridians of the legs are of fundamental importance in the management, transformation, and movement of fluids (and blood).

The Wrists

The wrists are the point of connection between the forearm and the hand. Through them, energy is expressed in an expressive way through the movement of the hands and fingers, or in a subtle way through various points, of which Lao gong (PC8) is the most important. If the wrists are blocked, energy cannot pass, art cannot take shape, it cannot manifest itself: whether it be music, graphic art, or craftsmanship, the wrist represents the path of fire, the creativity that can manifest itself. And in fact, on the wrist we find the yuan points of the heart, pericardium, triple heater, and small intestine: fire in all its forms.

The neck

The neck is a segment and passageway for our emotions, and when we experience discomfort in this area of the body, it means that there is a lack of balance between the parts involved and an inability to orient ourselves in the space around us.

What arises in the brain before we move passes through the neck, and this is specific to the gallbladder meridian, the energy channel of choices and directions to take.

If you have a disorder in this area, you are unable to orient yourself in the space of your life and you only look in one direction. You are unable to have a clear and "panoramic" view of your surroundings and therefore live without grasping the stimuli and opportunities around you, as if you were blindfolded.

In fact, pain in this area can often radiate to the eyes.

The local points that can allow movement and release tension are:

- SI.15 - SI.14 - VB.21

The distal points, on the other hand, are:

- IC.4 - IC.10 - IC.11

To be treated frequently throughout the day, repeating mentally:

I can move forward in life, I can choose, and if I make a mistake, I have learned something new. I am responsible, and therefore I CHOOSE!

The tongue and its reading to make a diagnosis

A very broad discussion should be had regarding the analysis of the tongue because it provides a great deal of information. Here, I will limit myself to reporting the most common and easily identifiable signs:

Red tongue (without coating): excess heat (and lack of fluids) – excess yang and yin deficiency

Tongue with a light coating: excess fluids and cold

Tongue with yellow coating: stomach heat with excess fluids

Tongue with teeth marks on the edges (and very moist): deficiency of spleen Qi (also deficiency of kidney yang)

Tongue that vibrates: internal wind, liver fire

184

Tongue cracked in the middle: stomach and constitutional deficiency

Tongue cracked to the tip: constitutional and heart (Shen) deficiency

Tongue with numerous cracks all over: kidney deficiency

Dark sublingual veins: liver Qi stagnation

Investigation

In order to understand people's characteristics, what their defining features are and therefore their critical points, the most delicate seasons, and the precautions they need to take to stay healthy, it is important to get to know the person according to the basic principles of Chinese medicine: Yin/Yang and the 5 movements. Through observation, but even more so through interviews with specific questions, it is possible to place the individual in a narrower portion of the infinite possibilities that can occur in nature. This is a complex task that requires knowledge and attention to the person. Strangely, however, modern Western medicine has established that all individuals are the same or at least very similar. Recently, more importance has been given to hormones as variables that disrupt the general rules, but this interpretation seems more like an excuse to confirm when a rule is disregarded in reality.

The principles are: seek fullness and emptiness

QUESTION: it is essential to listen to what the patient says and, above all, to the first things they say. Ask about their life and their ailments, where they feel pain or discomfort. Investigate primary and secondary symptoms (breathing, appetite, stools, urine, waking times, etc.) and their duration.

The energy diagnosis is used to understand which element or organ is most disturbed and to trace it back to the relative who is bothering them (mother-child cycle, grandparent-grandchild).

The etiology, or cause of the imbalance, is necessary to understand how the current illness arose and can be of two types:

-Exogenous (external): cold, heat, dryness, humidity, wind, and accidents

-Endogenous (internal): emotions and diet

-Mixed: for example, exposure to cold combined with poor nutrition

Fundamental relationship based on the relationship between yin and yang

186

-Cold or hot? That is, "do you prefer to be cold or hot?", "do you feel better in the heat or in the cold?", "do you suffer more from the cold or the heat?", "when you go out, are you more concerned about suffering from the heat or the cold"?

In the event of illness, it is important to know its origins, how it began, how it developed, how it reacts in terms of energy (hot/cold, drowsiness/agitation, etc.).

Therefore, it is crucial to identify which prevails: YIN or YANG?

But how should we intervene? According to some, we need to counteract the stronger polarity by introducing the weaker one. But this is not always correct because if, compared to the norm, the individual has an excess of Yin or Yang energy, it is more useful to discharge the excess rather than try to bring the other energy polarity into excess (which is highly unlikely). This is because the individual will naturally have their own level of balance, and when there is an excess, it is an exceptional situation that should not be maintained. Furthermore, it is clear that the excess is a temporary situation, so (for example, in the case of an excess of yang due to heatstroke or overeating) increasing Yin may have a temporary effect, but then Yin will naturally return to its normal state and, in fact, Yang, in order to counteract an artificially increased Yin, will consume it further, thus reducing Yin to a state of deficit and causing a further imbalance. Therefore, in the case of excess, it is always good to discharge what is in excess to restore balance and then, if the other polarity is deficient, strengthen it.

The case of deficit is different, where it is necessary to try to bring in the missing energy: a deficit of yin (such as sleep) rather than yang (cooling). The example of sleep is apt because it can happen that we are so exhausted that we become agitated and cannot fall asleep. It would seem to be an excess of yang, but if we check how yang the person really is (for example, by asking, 'Would you like to go for a run?'), the person would immediately feel the answer before even thinking about it: weakness in the legs, slouching posture... in short, the body would tell us what the mind might not say. On the other hand, a controversial yang deficiency could be constitutional and cause fluid retention, but according to current theories, you need to drink 2 liters of water a day. If the person were to follow this rule, they would feed the yin and suffocate the yang (water extinguishes fire, the fire needed to move and evaporate excess fluids), so if they really cannot help drinking, they should drink hot herbal teas, eat spicy foods, and thus bring yang into the body.

Pain, which is one of the indicators of a person's state of well-being or ill-being, can be classified according to the principles of Yin/Yang or based on energy lodges as follows

• Cold: chronic pain, excess YIN, relieved by heat

188

• Hot: acute pain, excess YANG, improves with cold

• Heavy: continuous and heavy pain, excess internal moisture, requires heat that moves but does not overheat

• Stinging: erratic pain that moves around, excess wind

• Chest pain: organic or energetic change in the heart or lungs

• Hypochondriac pain: liver and gallbladder

• Abdominal pain: from fullness (worsened by pressure, excess Yang) or emptiness (relieved by pressure, excess Yin)

• Headache: depends on location, for example, frontal pain represents the stomach and the earth element, in the temporal area the gallbladder and therefore wood, as well as wood if at the top of the head, but in this case it is the liver.

• Back pain: kidney deficiency, water element, as well as knee pain

• Muscle pain: earth element, probably excess moisture

• Pain when stretching rather than during muscular effort: wood element, therefore liver Qi stagnation

Other useful questions are:

-Breathing: do you have more discomfort when inhaling (kidney) or exhaling (lung)?

-Sweating: if you sweat easily, it is lung Qi deficiency; if you never sweat, it could be yin deficiency.

-Thirst: excessive (excess Yang), low (excess Yin)

-Appetite: no (spleen deficiency), yes (stomach or spleen fire)

-Stool: hard (excess heat), soft (excess cold, excess Yin) while constipation can occur in completely different situations:

• From heat: in the large intestine or stomach, with yellow, scanty urine, depletion of fluids

• From cold: Yin, large intestine deficiency, presenting with abundant urine

• Qi disorder: heaviness, pain, rumbling

• Qi deficiency: shortness of breath, asthenia. This condition is clearly related to the lungs because they are the organ that distributes Qi throughout the body, so if breathing is shallow, it is because there is a lack of Qi. asthenia is an indication of a lack of Qi, so constipation is probably caused by a lack of Qi that activates peristalsis (the amplitude of the diaphragm movement also contributes to this function), and we should remember that the lungs and large intestine belong to the same "movement": metal.

Diarrhea can also occur in different situations:

• Spleen deficiency: weak pulse, white tongue, feeling of oppression and fullness in the abdomen

190

• Cold and dampness: watery stools, abdominal pain, white nails

• Dampness and heat: abdominal pain, dark stools, burning sensation in the anus, yellow tongue

• Diet: imbalance of the stomach and spleen, abdominal pain, smell of rotten eggs due to irregular, excessive, or insufficient diet

• Kidney Qi deficiency: pain around the navel, intolerance to cold, cold lower limbs, right kidney deficiency (YANG)

Urine assessment gives us an indication of whether organic fluids are sufficient or insufficient (which are activated by lung and spleen Qi), and whether there is heat or cold.

Heat syndrome:

• Heat in the heart: dark yellow urine, associated with insomnia

• Liver and gallbladder heat: dark yellow urine, associated with pain in the hypochondria

• Stomach and large intestine heat: dark yellow urine associated with abdominal pain

Dark, yellow urine: excess Yang

Light urine: excess Yin, excess cold, pale tongue, hyperlaxity of the ligaments (in fact, when we are in the cold for a long time, it is easy to have to urinate several times precisely because the cold invades the bladder and the yang that holds the lower orifices is lacking.

Abundant and clear urine: Kidney yang deficiency

Abundant, clear urine, weak pulse, pale tongue: full of yin and internal cold

Incontinence: kidney qi deficiency

Sleep is also an element that can provide many clues.

• Heart YIN deficiency: palpitations, red tongue, insomnia

• Heart-Kidney axis imbalance: difficulty falling asleep, hyperlaxity of the knees, psychological breakdown

• Heart and spleen deficiency: light sleep, white tongue, weak pulse

• Dampness and phlegm: yellow tongue, excessive saliva, dizziness, chest tightness, nausea, feeling of fullness and heaviness in the head, headache: restless sleep

• Heat in the liver: dizziness, visual problems, nausea, irritability. If the heat increases, it can turn into fire: waking up at night with difficulty falling asleep.

It is important to pay attention if you wake up at night at the same times: from 1 a.m. to 3 a.m. is the liver time slot, from 3 a.m. to 5 a.m. is the lung time slot. From 5 a.m. to 7 a.m. is the large intestine time slot. If you wake up at these times, it means that those organs are affected. The liver with fire and agitation, the lungs with a Qi deficiency that worsens if you are unable to rest well. So if you start suffering from waking up between 3 and 5 a.m., you need to adopt strategies: either go to bed early to get enough sleep, or use products that promote sleep because the less you recharge your lung Qi, the less you recharge your Qi in general, and then you enter a vicious circle.

If you fall asleep easily in the evening, it is a yang deficiency, while if you wake up easily during the night and are unable to get back to sleep, it is a yin deficiency (yin brings us back to the resting phase).

I will now mention some of the most common disorders to draw attention to the various patterns of deficiency or excess that can be encountered when giving a practical energy reading:

Cold: obstruction of Lung Qi leading to aversion to cold or weakening of the lungs due to invasion by cold and wind. External pathogens weaken Lung Qi (especially in people with a Yin constitution).

Impotence: caused by a deficiency of kidney Qi, associated with low back pain and weakness in the knees

Hearing: the RIGHT ear is connected to the liver, liver fire, or excess moisture in the gallbladder; the LEFT ear is connected to the kidney, in particular corresponding to kidney Yin deficiency, with prolonged but intermittent tinnitus.

Nose: invasion of wind, which can be cold or hot, resulting in liquid, whitish mucus or thick, yellow/green mucus, respectively

Medical history

It is essential to take a medical history, gathering information about the family (family history) and the individual (personal history).

The personal medical history consists of questions about hobbies, addictions, diet, etc. (e.g., asking what flavor they prefer, as each flavor is connected to an organ; in fact, we have salty connected to the kidney, sweet to the spleen, bitter to the heart, spicy to the lung, and sour to the liver).

During this phase, it is important to observe the person to see their non-verbal signs, to see their Shen, their vitality, their Qi, their Essence, their Xue, and the energetic state of their organs.

Look at the person's pupils, see how they move. If they remain abnormally and excessively fixed, there is probably a deficiency; if they move frantically, there is probably an excess or wind.

If vitality is strong, prenatal Kidney Qi is strong, the organs are good, the eyes are bright, the skin is radiant, and the voice is semi-loud.

When vitality is lacking, the Jing of the kidneys is weak, perhaps depleted, the gaze is empty, and there is general asthenia. If the voice is weak, there is weakness of Lung Qi.

Observing the color of the skin directs us to the organ (energy lodge) that is suffering:

red, blue, green, white, yellow, and black depending on the affected organ.

These colors are very clearly expressed in the face, which is closely related to the abdomen. In particular, blue represents blood stasis, an invasion of cold wind, or an excess of yin and cold. The color red is caused by an excess of internal heat, particularly in the heart or small intestine. This coloration is normal in summer, but not in other seasons (summer being the season associated with the fire lodge).

A red coloration at the cheekbones represents an excess of yang or a deficiency of yin. When a person has a pale complexion that turns red, we have an excess of yang.

The color yellow is a symptom of fatigue and excess moisture, associated with a deficiency of spleen qi.

A white face, on the other hand, represents cold, asthenia, and Lung Qi that is unable to properly diffuse Qi to move the blood.

Finally, a dark face is indicative of an excess of yin and a deficiency of the kidneys, both right and left.

It is clear that there are many distinctive signs that can give us indications of what is in excess and what is deficient, far more than those indicated above, but starting to have clear and well-directed indications serves as a compass to begin to focus attention on certain elements, connect them to energy lodges or energy polarities, and from there begin to intervene. Or, simply, to know oneself and know one's neighbor, which is already a good starting point. It is not always possible to implement change, but removing the label of 'sick' or avoiding judgments that serve no one (except in some cases to worsen the situation) and highlighting a new level of awareness of the person's nature can only serve to observe with the right detachment and without judgment. It is then the will of the individual (kidney) that can trigger the desire for change, or for acceptance and peace with oneself.

The vagus nerve: a channel unto itself

Humans have an autonomic nervous system that is actually composed of three separate subsystems:

the parasympathetic nervous system (PNS) - Yin

the sympathetic nervous system (SNS) - Yang

the enteric nervous system (ENS)

The enteric nervous system has been described as a "second brain," which communicates with the central nervous system (CNS) through the parasympathetic (e.g., via the vagus nerve) and sympathetic nervous systems.

However, studies on vertebrates show that when the vagus nerve is severed, the enteric nervous system continues to function.

We now know that the ENS not only has autonomy but also influences the brain.

In fact, about 90 percent of the signals that pass along the vagus nerve do not come from above, but from the ENS, which is why many consider it to be a backup brain centered in our solar plexus.

Our visceral instincts are not fantasies but real nerve signals that guide much of our lives.

It is our vagus nerve that provides the gateway between the two parts of the autonomic systems.

The vagus acts as a bioinformative data bus that routes impulses in two directions.

Since the vagus nerve acts as a switchboard, it should come as no surprise that impaired functioning of this nerve can lead to so many different conditions and problems.

Some neurological diseases actually originate in the gut and spread to the brain via the vagus nerve.

The autonomic nervous system is composed of two opposing polar systems that create a complementary tug-of-war, allowing the body to maintain homeostasis (inner stability).

The sympathetic nervous system is designed to rev you up like the accelerator pedal in a car: it feeds on adrenaline and cortisol and is part of the "fight or flight" response.

The parasympathetic nervous system is the exact opposite. The vagus nerve is the command center for parasympathetic nervous system function.

Unfortunately, the reflexive responses of the vagus nerve can backfire and turn it from a companion into a saboteur.

The vagus nerve is known as the "wandering nerve" because it has multiple branches that diverge from two thick stems rooted in the cerebellum and brainstem, wandering down to the lower viscera of our abdomen, touching our heart and most of the major organs along the way.

Vagus means "wandering" in Latin.

It winds its way down to the belly, spreading fibers to the tongue, pharynx, vocal cords, lungs, heart, stomach, intestines, and glands that produce enzymes and anti-stress hormones (such as acetylcholine, prolactin, vasopressin, oxytocin), affecting digestion, metabolism, and the response to relaxation.

The vagus nerve reaches the genitals, and therefore sexuality is directly involved in its functioning (and vice versa). If our brain cannot communicate with the diaphragm through the release of acetylcholine from the vagus nerve, we will stop breathing (Botox is a toxic substance that has the power to damage the nervous system and deactivate the vagus nerve, causing its death).

The vagus nerve is one of the largest nervous systems in the body.

The vagus is used to send a variety of signals throughout the body, but it also transfers signals to the brain. The vagus nerve constantly sends updated sensory information about the state of the body's organs "upstream" to the brain via the afferent nerves.

In fact, 80-90% of the nerve fibers in the vagus nerve are dedicated to communicating the status of the viscera to the brain. The vagus nerve helps manage the complex processes of the digestive tract, including signaling the stomach muscles to contract and push food into the small intestine.

A damaged vagus nerve cannot send signals to the stomach muscles. This can cause food to remain in the stomach longer, rather than moving normally into the small intestine to be digested. Because the vagus nerve provides parasympathetic motor fibers to all organs from the neck to the second segment of the transverse colon (except the adrenal glands), its effect can be far-reaching.

Stress can increase the level of epinephrine and norepinephrine in the body, which stimulate the sympathetic nervous system to prevail over the parasympathetic nervous system, of which the vagus nerve is the main component.

The vagus nerve is used to regulate heartbeat and the muscle movement necessary to maintain breathing.

This nerve also regulates chemical levels in the digestive system so that the intestines can process food and keep track of what types of nutrients are obtained from the food ingested.

There are two main types of vagus nerve disorders. One is caused by an underactive or inactive vagus nerve, while the other is caused by a vagus nerve that overreacts to ordinary stimuli.

Vagus nerve disorders that result from a hypoactive vagus nerve often lead to a condition known as gastroparesis, a common and serious complication of diabetes. Patients suffering from this disorder may experience stomach pain, nausea, heartburn, stomach spasms, and weight loss.

Patients with hypoactive vagus nerves often have severe gastrointestinal problems. Those with hyperactive vagus nerves may faint.

200

Any type of gastrointestinal disorder can put pressure on the nerve and irritate it. Poor posture combined with muscle imbalances can also cause the vagus nerve to fail to fire, as can stress combined with fatigue and anxiety. Many people who experience symptoms of vagal dysfunction have what in Chinese medicine might be described as a gallbladder and heart complex.

This has traditionally been a diagnosis used to describe a set of symptoms such as esophagitis, hiatal hernia, gastritis, insomnia, palpitations, fear, easily frightened, chest fullness, and bitter taste in the mouth. In these people, access to the divergent channel of the gallbladder can bring almost immediate relief.

In concrete terms:

-        Stimulate GB 30 and GB 1 with acupressure, along with GB 34, LIV 3, PC6, SP 4, LIV 14, and GB 19.

-        Moving and stretching can also relieve pressure and act on the vagus nerve.

-        Massage the upper part of the ear, rubbing it until it turns red.

-        Herbs that stimulate digestion (Emblica, Milk Thistle)

-        Herbs capable of regulating the neuroendocrine system (all primary adaptogens)

-        Hold your breath and lower your diaphragm

- Immerse your face in ice water (immersion reflex)

- Coughing (exercises a mechanical action that reaches the vagus nerve)

- Laugh heartily (same as above)

- Belching (same as above)

Similarly, diaphragmatic breathing, physical activity, and meditation help the parasympathetic nervous system prevail over the sympathetic nervous system and regulate vagal function, thereby initiating the tissue regeneration process that we can refer to as the "Yin phase," which occurs mainly during sleep.

The vagus nerve also plays a regulatory role in the expression of emotions, controlling states such as fear and giving us the ability to maintain control in extreme situations.

9.2 Eight diagnostic rules

In the previous paragraph, we deliberately took a more scientific approach to understanding ourselves. The subject is vast and can be addressed using many different methodologies. The more you know, the more likely you are to get confused if you are not a professional with extensive theoretical training and field experience. For this reason, according to the Chinese medicine approach, individual energetic or physiological conditions can be identified by applying a few basic rules. Always remember Pareto's law: with 80% of quantitative data, you obtain 20% of qualitative data and vice versa. Therefore, even with only 20% of the qualitative data, you can obtain 80% of the quantitative data, which determines almost the entirety of the individual. Thus, by using the concepts of the five movements and the eight diagnostic rules, you can almost completely frame a temporary and long-term (constitutional) condition of the individual. The eight diagnostic rules are:

- Yin/Yang: discussed in chapter 3

- Full/Empty: discussed in chapter 5

- Hot / Cold: which, for simplicity's sake, we can trace back to the Yin / Yang rule

- Internal/External: this is a more professional approach, but we can summarize it with the causes that lead to an im r imbalance. Therefore, external causes are effects that come from outside, such as climatic effects, viruses, and nutrition, while internal causes are everything that is emotional or connected to a weakness or malfunction of an energy lodge.

When we correctly answer these four questions about the causes of what has caused us a disorder (whether temporary or chronic, if not constitutional), we will already understand which path we are on and will have all the tools we need to decide whether to stay on that path or change course. This compendium will not provide all the solutions, but it can be a compass to guide us in seeking solutions elsewhere: a specific professional (acupuncturist, nutritionist, personal trainer, etc.), a manual (phytotherapy, Qigong, dietetics, etc.) or any other source that may be useful to us. Having gained awareness will enable us to keep our antennae up and better receive the input that will surely come from outside.

10. THE ENCOUNTER BETWEEN EAST AND WEST

10.1 Chinese medicine in the Western context

All too often we hear that Eastern practices are not suitable for Westerners for cultural reasons, because they are based on folklore, because they are not scientific... in short: a series of excuses are sought so as not to attribute to them the authority that allowed these disciplines to emerge between 4,000 and

5,000 years ago, to be perfected over the centuries and to arrive at the present day while maintaining the roots and principles already known a few millennia ago. A little common sense would suffice to admit that if knowledge exists and has been preserved for so long, it certainly has foundations and bases that are unquestionably more tested than Western sciences, which have only developed in the last two centuries, making giant strides in specialization and hyperspecialization, in micron-level investigation and in surgery, but precisely because of this hyperspecialization and the pursuit of point analysis, it has very often lost sight of the whole. Fortunately, many Western scientists have come across these disciplines and have managed to identify points of contact, translating the energy diagnoses of Eastern medicine into Western pathologies, inventing PNEI, etc.

Western medicine is certainly extremely effective in emergencies (i.e., topical symptoms, surgery, etc.), while Eastern medicine should be recognized as a rule of healthy living to maintain good health or restore energy balance in the event of illness or chronic disease. Eastern medicine tends not to have immediate effects— but this is not always true, as acupuncture and herbal medicine can be effective after just a few treatments, which means within a week or two at most—but since they are "disciplines," they should be read more as instruction manuals for using our body, mind, and spirit well. There is no interest in discrediting 'the other science', as the Western mainstream and, in many cases, Western medicine itself, seek to do. This type of approach is short-sighted and harmful to the individual because it prevents them from being properly monitored and treated by a specialist who studies them in their entirety in order to provide them with instructions suited to their nature, constitution, age, gender, etc. This is to the advantage of a method that standardizes pathologies and treatments, as if we were all identical machines that suffer from disorders for a single reason and can only receive one type of treatment that produces the same effects on everyone.

You don't need a degree in biology to understand that this approach is totally nonsensical... yet for decades they have wanted us to believe that this is the case. So the only sensible thing we can do to stay healthy, or rather, is not to delegate the care of ourselves to others. Let's eat well, follow the rules of healthy living, exercise, get the right amount of sleep, and yes, take the medicine we need when we need it. For the rest, nature has provided us with all the tools we need to stay healthy; we just have to want to do it. Because let's remember that, whether we are healthy or sick... we are the only ones who benefit or suffer from the difference between these two conditions. So we must take back this responsibility that the Western approach of "a spoonful of sugar helps the medicine go down" has taken away from us, because it requires less effort.

10.2 Integrating the principles of Chinese medicine into modern life

We have reviewed many principles of Chinese medicine—yin, yang, the five movements, Qigong, breathing—to reawaken knowledge that belongs to us (if we look closely, Hippocrates did not talk about very different things). The purpose of this overview is to learn to read ourselves as if we were a map: once we know the meanings of the symbols, we can recognize the individual elements, understand what makes us feel good and what makes us feel bad, what we need and what we can do without. Not to have control over everything, but to have more freedom of expression. If we know ourselves, we can make the most of our abilities, increase them, limit the depletion of the resources we have little of, and so on. Know thyself is a Greek motto, not a Chinese one, yet the principle is universal: through Chinese medicine diagnosis, you are already halfway to healing and good health.

We must not adapt to other people's lifestyles because, although we may be able to adapt for a short period of time, certain behaviors could prove extremely harmful to us in the long run. Some people are lucky (genetically, Jing) enough not to have cholesterol problems even though they don't exercise and eat foods rich in fat. But it is unlikely that I will be as lucky. Certainly, maintaining a lifestyle consisting of a proper and balanced diet, physical activity, rest, study, social life, and meditation can only benefit me and keep my energy levels moderately high. Illness or disorder can happen, but if it affects me and my energy reserves are low, I will certainly have more difficulty reacting, healing, and recovering. We need to think about this. This does not mean depriving ourselves of everything, but not overdoing it. Enjoying life with a few moments of excess if it happens and if we feel it makes us feel good is fine, as this can also nourish our Shen, but precisely because it is not a rule or a habit, which then becomes almost a slavery to an unnatural lifestyle that depletes our energy and makes us ugly as human beings.

In spring, the cycle of nature begins again, awakening, the sap begins to circulate again to bring new energy to living beings so that they can grow, expand, and generate. But often this movement of expansion is blocked, constrained, or lacks energy because the liver (the organ of wood movement) is clogged with toxins: physical and emotional. The liver must purify the blood, and during winter, as we use up all our resources, residues, dense matter, and waste remain. If the liver is too clogged, it struggles to release energy and becomes overwhelmed, leading to excessive anger, exhaustion even after resting, neck pain, and digestive difficulties. The main action to take is purification through drinks and herbal teas (dandelion, lemon, turmeric, artichoke), but also purification from negative emotions, so calm your anger, take walks (the liver likes walking) in green spaces (the color of wood movement).

In summer, long days lead people to be more active and high temperatures lead to fluid consumption. The effect of these elements, if there is no control and awareness of one's resources, leads to excessive consumption of Qi and weakening, which will cause susceptibility to illness in autumn. It is important to drink, including isotonic drinks, to replenish the loss of mineral salts that occurs with sweating. Sweating is good for you, as it helps eliminate toxins, whereas air conditioning actually closes the pores of the skin and retains toxins. Eat fresh, lightly spiced foods and, if you tend to sweat a lot, add lemon or grapefruit to your drinks: the acid retains fluids and prevents excessive loss.

Late summer—the season associated with earth movement—is the time when you can engage in more intense physical exercise because the climate is favorable and the body is full of energy. It is important to strengthen muscles, drain fluids, and promote circulation to replace the old with the new, renewing the blood (which occurs through hematopoiesis: working on the spleen and washing the marrow – Qigong and taiji exercises).

Autumn is the season when daylight begins to decline and cold winds arrive, affecting the respiratory system by attacking the epidermis (the lungs are connected to the skin). Astragalus, which supports the immune system, and ginger, which stimulates and is slightly spicy, are highly recommended. It is always important to drink hot or warm beverages, exercise, and above all breathe deeply because, in addition to emptying the lungs to renew them, the movement of deep breathing aids peristalsis and therefore the elimination of waste from the large intestine (connected to the lungs). In this season, we slow down and observe ourselves.

Winter is the season of rest: fewer hours of daylight means fewer hours of activity. We should also accept the cold, both to slow down our pace and to avoid being affected by excessive temperature changes. The temperature in the home should not exceed 20 degrees. We should accept that we need to rest more, sleep more, relax more, meditate more, and not overdo sport, especially in the evening, which is a time for rest. In any case, sport should not involve excessive sweating and fat consumption, which we naturally need to combat the seasonal cold. Colds are fought with rest, steam inhalation (not boiling water, otherwise it dries out the mucus), vitamin C, astragalus, echinacea, and honey. Let the illness run its course so that our body is trained to win the battle, with the support of the right foods, without rushing to 'do', 'produce' or 'get back on the merry-go-round': the world will go on without us for a few days and it is better to regenerate completely than to return to the fray still aching or with low batteries (our yin and yang kidneys).

10.3 Dietetics

Dietetics covers a very broad chapter within Chinese medicine, certainly broader than acupuncture itself, and represents a cornerstone for people's health. After all, nutrition accounts for 50% of who we are, i.e., wh s we ingest are assimilated, or made similar to ourselves based on our genetic heritage, and transformed into the substantial part of ourselves. Then there is what we breathe, there are emotions, there is what we do, but the substance comes from food. Dedicating a single paragraph to dietetics is not to belittle it, but rather to avoid delving too deeply into a subject that has been dealt with by so many, a subject that has been so popular in recent decades that so many forms and formulas of diets have arisen that it has probably caused more confusion than education on the subject.

Therefore, in line with the purpose of this book, we intend to summarize the principles by providing practical instructions and a systemic approach to nutrition. It should also be noted that herbal medicine is a different practice, even more targeted and specific, aimed at treating pathological conditions, and therefore short-term, while dietetics aims at preservation, maintenance, growth, and correction, but with a long-term perspective.

First of all, according to Chinese medicine, when eating, attention should be paid to what you eat. It is also a social occasion, so it is important to pay attention to the food, flavors, colors, and arrangement of the food and the table (feng shui). Then you need to be calm when you sit down to eat: your heart must be calm and your stomach must be well disposed. You need to sit with your back straight so as not to compress your stomach and allow food to pass through easily. Your stomach should be half full of food, a quarter full of water and a quarter full of air, so you need to leave the table with enough space to be active and not overwhelmed by food and drink. It is best to settle the stomach with warm or lukewarm food so as not to consume too much yang for digestion or block the stomach, especially in cold seasons or on cold days. Cold weather extinguishes the yang in the stomach, which is needed to transform food. Too much heat, on the other hand, can cause stomach fire. In the evening, it is good to spend at least 2-3 hours awake before going to sleep, and in any case, after each meal, it is advisable to take 100 steps—which means moving, walking, standing, without fatigue or effort, but maintaining movement to circulate Qi and, thanks to movement, promote peristalsis. Furthermore, "Not eating when hungry and not drinking when thirsty depletes the source of Qi and blood production, weakens the organs, and causes illness. Not eating for half a day weakens the Qi for one day and diminishes it for eight days, emptying the Qi of the stomach." And again, "Eating too much constantly causes premature aging, especially for those who work with their minds.".

Obviously, foods must be chosen to balance personal and environmental excesses and imbalances. In winter, it is good to eat foods that warm you up and are hot, to nourish the yang y . In summer, it is good to drink and eat fresh foods, but you must be careful not to overdo it because the fire must be reduced but not extinguished (it is more risky to eat food that is too cold than food that is too hot).

From the point of view of the elements, or movements, individuals should always try not to eat foods with excessive characteristics but remain within a medium range. What does this mean?

In dietetics, each food has its own energetic characteristic—corresponding to the five movements—which is given by its flavor. So, based on its flavor, a food will be: sour (wood), bitter (fire), sweet (earth), spicy (metal), salty (water). In addition to flavor, nature also counts: hot, cold, warm, cool. Let's say that in a non-pathological condition, it is fine to eat warm or cool foods with mild flavors. In the case of pathologies, even chronic ones, the focus will be on hot or cold foods and more pronounced flavors.

In dietetics, more than in other disciplines of Chinese medicine, it is essential to nourish the center, i.e., the earth, stomach, and spleen. The stomach is the granary of the organs, so it must function well because it is the source of the nourishment that will then be transformed and transported by the blood to the various organs that will be nourished. In fact, in the case of illness, boiled rice (even very well cooked) is always recommended to restore energy to the earth.

In the case of acute pathology, one should seek the flavor that most nourishes the energy lodge involved. But how? The flavor mentioned above nourishes and rebalances the lodge, or, starting from a classic text that reads

"....What wets and descends (water) is salty, what blazes upwards (fire) is bitter, what can be bent and straightened (wood) is sour, what can be shaped and tempered (metal) is spicy, what allows sowing and growth (earth) is sweet." "Shang Shu" ZHOU Dynasty (1000-771 BC).

Three flavors are yin (they increase yin characteristics): sour, salty, bitter

Two flavors are yang (increase yang characteristics): sweet, spicy.

Wood: sour astringes, retains, condenses, which is good for the liver, which risks expanding too much due to too much fire (anger, rage), or because it tends to invade, being made up of blood, and therefore must be contained because, if there is no rooting in the blood, the hun (the ethereal spirit) disperses. Excess causes Qi and Qini stagnation, cramps, and muscle contractions.

Fire: bitter purifies and brings down, which is good for containing a blazing fire, for a heart that risks becoming excited and having a heart attack, for a Shen that seeks to return to the great Shen, to the one, and therefore leave the body. Excess slows down energy and blocks expansion, causing contractions and vomiting.

Earth: sweet, but without exaggeration, balances, stabilizes, contains all the elements and prevents them from dispersing. Excess obstructs distribution, creating stagnation (of liquids or food).

Metal: spicy, to move and expand, the opposite of wood, because metal, the lungs, risk collapsing in on themselves when they should be moving outward to feel alive and not get stuck. Excess can also disperse Qi through sweating.

Water: salty, which brings down and softens, it is a mild saltiness. Excess softens the flesh and energy is unstructured.

Three flavors are yin (they increase yin characteristics): sour, salty, bitter

Two flavors are yang (increase yang characteristics): sweet and spicy.

In case of excess, however, the flavor of the child will be used, i.e., in case of excess fire, sweet will be used to weaken the mother.

In the case of deficiency in chronic diseases, on the other hand, the mother will be nourished so that she can nourish the child. The strategy of nourishing the mother is recommended in chronic diseases because a long-term balance must be established. Therefore, if the child is deficient, it is probably because they have not received the right nourishment from the mother, so we must start with the mother to strengthen her and thus strengthen the child.

Therefore, returning to the main laws of movement, we have that

According to the law of generation:

acid (Wood) nourishes the liver and heart,

bitter (Fire) nourishes the heart and spleen,

sweet (Earth) nourishes the spleen and lungs,

spicy (Metal) nourishes the lungs and kidneys

Salt (water) nourishes the kidneys and liver.

According to the law of control-domination:

sour dominates the spleen and balances sweet flavor

bitter dominates the lungs and balances spicy

sweet dominates the kidneys and balances saltiness

spicy dominates the liver and balances sour.

salty dominates the heart and balances bitter.

At this point, it is appropriate to give specific information on the characteristics of foods, starting with their nature:

Hot nature:

creates heat, warms the interior and organs in yang weakness, it is a property of extreme remedies (aconite, cinnamon, dried ginger). The stomach, liver, and heart suffer most from internal heat.

Warm nature:

dispels cold and yin fullness (brown rice, oats, green beans, pumpkin, onion, bell pepper, leek, carrot, chicken, sheep's cheese, sheep's milk, lamb, wild boar, tripe, chicken livers, cherry, coconut, date, jujube, raspberry, peach, apricot, quince, walnuts, pine nuts, parsley, dill, basil, rosemary, thyme, ginger, capers, nutmeg, maltose, brown sugar, red vinegar, wine, anchovies, shrimp, mackerel, lobster, mussels, squid...)

Cold nature:

creates cold, cools the organs, calms fire, detoxifies, disperses yang fullness (watermelon, tomato, seaweed, banana). The spleen, kidney, stomach, and uterus are particularly sensitive to cold.

Cool nature:

reduces heat (wheat, barley, chard, eggplant, turnip, radish, lettuce, spinach, celery, soybeans, egg white, butter, rabbit, lard, octopus, cow's milk, frog, horse, snail, duck, apple, pear, melon, tangerine, plum, orange, lemon, marjoram, mint, oregano, tea, sesame oil, brown sugar, salt, soy sauce, crab, oyster...)

The cooking method affects the nature of food: it is necessary, but the characteristics of vitality must be maintained. Cooking is also necessary to vary the extreme characteristics:

- baking or stewing increases heat (mitigates cold nature),

- frying adds a lot of heat, can dry out liquids, and is toxic (ginger)

- grilling heats and dries (good for vegetables but not for hot meats)

- boiling decreases the nature (cools),

- steaming or bain-marie cooking does not alter it and increases digestibility.

- Microwaving alters the nature and has a drying effect.

- Stir-frying (wok) maintains characteristics, makes food more digestible, and energizes.

- Sautéing with ginger or alcohol increases the ability to move

- Stir-frying with vinegar and/or honey moisturizes it and makes it more yin.

Moving on now to the discussion of flavors (some foods codified by Chinese dietetics will be mentioned, which may not be considered customary or appropriate to our culture):

ACIDIC - wood-liver:

a moderate flavor moisturizes and nourishes the yin of the liver. Excess disperses the energy of the liver and spleen, damaging muscles, tendons, and connective tissue. It acts on the nerves, limiting chronic pain. Action on energy: the liver distributes Qi in all directions, acid can collect, astringe, and contract. It facilitates all evacuations. In excess of internal or external heat, it cools by concentrating yin, reducing the dispersion of fluids. When excessive, it can cause cramps and colic. Acidic foods: wheat, yeast, rye, tomato, sorrel, leek, spinach, azuki beans, peas, rabbit, chicken, egg yolk, dog, vinegar, lemon, yogurt, goat cheese, plum, pineapple, raspberry, orange, tangerine, strawberry, currant

BITTER- fire-heart:

-brings down, drains downwards (purgatives) all accumulations of food, heat, liquids, regulates the downward movement of Qi (QIni), dries liquids, dries what is damp. Bitter is warming, stimulates yang and counteracts excess yin by drying, calms: subtle bitter nourishes the yin of the heart, calms fire, excess disperses the energy of the heart and lungs, dries the skin , causes hair loss, stops heat hemorrhages, hardens, acts on the bones (avoid in bone diseases). Bitter foods: buckwheat, wheat, chicory, endive, cucumber, artichoke, shallots, asparagus, mutton, goat, pheasant, guinea fowl, game, liver, thyme, rosemary, sage, gentian, coffee, tea, apricot, grapefruit, loquat, bitter orange,

SWEET - earth-spleen:

subtle sweetness nourishes the yin of the spleen, harmonizes (licorice is the quintessential flavor of this food), tones energy and blood (rice), stops pain, and moisturizes. It acts on the muscles; excess causes muscle weakness. Sweet foods: rice, barley, red millet, corn, yeast, pumpkin, carrot, potato, zucchini, Jerusalem artichoke, fennel, peas, beef, heart, white fish, butter, cream, milk, fresh cow's milk cheese, oil, sugar, honey, sesame, jujube, banana, apple, grape, persimmon, date, fig, melon, (almost all fruit is sweet).

SPICY-metal-lung:

subtle spiciness nourishes lung yin, activates dispersing function, the lung governs the skin, induces sweating (eliminates external pathogens), circulates energy and blood, moves, aids digestion, straightens energy (cough), goes high and to the surface, disperses Qi (do not overdo in Qi voids).Spicy foods: oats, yellow millet, garlic, onion, leek, radish, watercress, , parsley, turnip, pepper, celery, eggplant, horse, chicken, pecorino cheese, pepper, paprika, ginger, mint, mustard, mustard sauce, (most spices), peach, walnuts, medlar, almond, citron, quince.

SALT – kidney-water:

Salty foods nourish kidney yin, but when consumed in excess they disperse energy, are harmful to bones, moisturize, soften hardness, dissolve accumulations, bring down internal accumulations, calm the spirit, and pacify internal wind. Excessive consumption can dry the blood and should be avoided in cases of blood deficiency. Salty foods: dried beans, soybeans, lentils (dried legumes), cabbage, savoy cabbage, cauliflower, lettuce, mushrooms, seaweed, pork, blue fish, seafood, asparagus, chestnuts.

Finally, there are three intermediate flavors, which are:

Bland: mildly sweet, stimulates diuresis (white rice)

Astringent: reduces loss of body fluids.

Aromatic: stimulates digestion, transforms moisture, helps the spleen; consumed when cooked.

Food should be in tune with the climate and season, and should be rich in Jing. The primary recommendations would be to:

-prefer local and seasonal products,

-fresh, unpreserved,

-varied in the 5 flavors,

-not overcooked but not raw

-and above all, eaten with joy.

As for food combinations, as mentioned above, in the West we have seen countless dietary theories and diets emerge in recent decades, many of which can be attributed to passing fads followed by the sale of products branded according to the type of diet. Apart from this, Western culture has focused its attention on micronutrients, classifying foods according to their carbohydrate, fat, sugar, and calorie content, etc., without taking into account their energy value, as we have listed above. For this reason, in Chinese dietetics, attention is focused primarily on energy and nature and, secondarily, on nutritional values. In fact, the guidelines for a proper meal are:

cereals should make up 50-60% of the meal,

meat should make up 10-20%,

fruit should make up 10-20%,

complementary foods and fillers, vegetables 20-30%.

This completely overturns the quantitative approach and shifts the focus to quality which, as mentioned at the beginning, is not only determined by the food and the combination of foods, but also by the way in which we approach the meal, the attention we pay to it, and the time we devote to digestion after the meal.

To conclude the discussion on dietetics, we will focus on the analysis of the individual's constitution in relation to nutrition. In fact, in addition to eating in accordance with what grows in their geographical area, based on the season and temperature, each of us should eat according to our own constitution. At this point in the discussion, you will be ready to "classify" yourself into a physical and metabolic type. Each individual has an energetic constitution that comes from the anterior sky. It indicates their tendency to become ill in a certain way, not a pathology.

Various classifications are possible, but for our purposes it is useful to think in terms of Yin-Yang.

Yin constitution: characterized by cold, dampness, yang deficiency

Yang constitution: characterized by heat, dryness, empty heat

YIN CONSTITUTION:

prevalence of yin and absolute or relative deficiency of yang; tends to stagnation of cold, dampness, and mucus. Main signs: sensitivity to cold, paleness, cold extremities and fear of cold, lack of energy, swollen body with a feeling of heaviness, tendency to be overweight or obese, succulence to the point of edema, loose stools to the point of chronic diarrhea, tendency to cystitis and vaginitis. The tongue is pale, swollen, indented, with a white coating; the pulse is slow and deep.

Avoid foods that are cool or cold in nature and have a strong sweet, sour, or salty taste, as these tend to further damage the weakened yang. Exclude foods that are difficult to digest, raw foods, and ice cream, which develop dampness, cold, and mucus. Prefer warm foods and, in moderation, hot foods; favor mildly sweet foods that tone, spicy foods that warm and stimulate, and bitter foods that dry moisture, depending on which of the three aspects prevails: cold, dampness, or yang deficiency.

COLD CONSTITUTION:

characterized by coldness, preference for hot drinks, paleness, asthenia, apathy, loss of appetite, and bloated abdomen, polyuria with clear urine, loose stools. It is recommended to warm up with warm foods that are sweet or spicy in flavor: leeks, shallots, sweet potatoes, turnips, onions, green beans, ganoderma mushrooms, pumpkin, asparagus , carrots, glutinous rice, brown rice, oats; mutton, chicken, lamb, shrimp, anchovies, mackerel, lobster, mussels; cherries, peaches, walnuts, lychees; spices; basil, dill, cloves, rosemary, thyme, fresh ginger, chives; maltose, brown sugar; red vinegar, red wine; sunflower oil, soybean oil. Foods that tone Qi (mutton, shrimp, prawns, walnuts) should be cooked with the addition of spices that tone yang, such as sage, garlic, anise, basil, cinnamon, cloves, fenugreek, nutmeg, rosemary, fennel seeds, thyme, and dried ginger. Prolonged cooking, roasting, and baking increase the warm quality of foods—do not overheat foods, especially spicy ones, which cause sweating and dispersion of Qi through perspiration. The process of strengthening yang must be gradual and requires time and consistency. Remember that yang needs yin. Avoid excessive consumption of foods and beverages that are cold in nature and temperature and bitter in taste.

WET CONSTITUTION:

Feeling of heaviness in the body, abdominal distension, moist tongue, overweight (due to fluid retention, fat, especially in the lower part of the body, e.g., cellulite), lack of thirst, asthenia. The constitutional tendency is aggravated by humid weather or a sedentary lifestyle. The tongue is swollen and marked. Diuresis should be promoted with bland-tasting, neutral foods: rice, azuki beans, corn, Job's tears, sunflower oil, sole, grifola, watercress, ginger peel, frog, sardines, clams, laminaria seaweed, green soybeans, lettuce, fenugreek, papaya, pineapple, alfalfa. For moisture in the intestines, basmati rice with basil, thyme, fennel, pumpkin; corn on the cob (make an infusion with the husks and fresh leaves for moisture in the bladder). If moisture is in the liver and gallbladder, the following are recommended: chicory, endive, rye, roasted barley, green soybeans with seaweed, barley with cabbage, fresh purslane, gentian, and dandelion. The transformation of moisture should be promoted with aromatic herbs that activate the function of the spleen: broad beans, garlic, cardamom, coriander, nutmeg, porcini mushrooms, fresh ginger, bay leaves, rosemary, basil; it is advisable to warm with lukewarm and spicy foods: turnips, radish, spring onion, pepper, leek, shallot, onion, kumquat, horseradish, dill, basil, parsley. You should also avoid excessive sweet and sour foods such as fruit juices, especially cold ones (mandarin is less cold); yogurt, dairy products, goat's and sheep's cheese cause less dampness because they are warm; Beer moistens more than wine (red wine is better). Avoid sugar and sweeteners, bananas, and animal fats. To dry moisture with heat, green soybeans are good. If it is moisture without heat, Job's tears (toasted in infusion) are good. Lukewarm jasmine green tea and Bojenmi tea stimulate both transformation and drainage away from meals. Shanyao (yam) diascorea. Rice is better than pasta; reduce bread and especially yeast, which creates dampness ( ), preferably toasted. Eat little fruit (preferably cooked with spices) and raw vegetables (preferably grilled). Be careful to avoid all dietary excesses, especially in the evening.

YANG DEFICIENCY CONSTITUTION:

physical and mental asthenia prevails, excessive perspiration even at rest and more during the day than at night, palpitations, shortness of breath, loss of appetite, possible organ ptosis. Pale

226

tongue. The deficiency (which is physiological with age) can be controlled with foods that are moderately sweet, salty (nourishes the kidneys), and warm, which tone energy, yang, and blood: rice, oats, dates, meat, fish, walnuts, and pistachios. Avoid foods that disperse energy, such as spicy foods that make you sweat and bitter foods; exclude foods that are cold in nature, excess fluids, raw and cold foods. Yang-tonifying foods: walnuts (3-4 per day), dried ginger, cinnamon bark in small quantities to ignite the mingmen fire, turmeric, nutmeg, capers, star anise, fennel seeds.

YANG CONSTITUTION

is characterized by a relative deficiency of yin, symptoms of heat (absolute or relative) and dryness. The main signs are: thinness, restlessness, irritability, aggressiveness, never tired, eats a lot but does not gain weight, red face, red eyes, fears heat, dresses lightly, constipation. The tongue is red with little yellow coating and cracks. It is necessary to avoid excessively warm, hot, bitter, and spicy foods because they consume fluids and substances that induce diuresis (dryness). Prefer foods that are neutral, fresh, or cold in nature and have a sour (produces fluids), moderately sweet, and salty taste. We distinguish three subtypes depending on whether heat, dryness, or yin deficiency prevails

HOT CONSTITUTION:

reddened face, burning red eyes (liver), burning and bleeding of the mucous membranes, scant and hyperchromic urine, hard stools with difficulty in passing. Tongue with yellow coating, rapid pulse. To balance excessive heat, foods that are cool in nature and sweet or bitter in taste should be consumed: wheat, millet, bamboo and soy sprouts, green soybeans, seaweed, Swiss chard, eggplant, tofu, cucumbers, melon, watermelon, grapefruit, lemon, banana, tea, chrysanthemum flower infusions (red eyes), asparagus, elderberry (jam or flower infusion), lettuce, egg white, peppermint. Avoid warm foods such as meat, shellfish, dried fruit, chocolate, coffee; avoid spicy foods and alcohol.

DRY CONSTITUTION:

symptoms include thirst, dry lips, nose, throat, skin, dry cough, itchy skin, possibly constipation and oliguria. It is necessary to moisturize and produce fluids with vegetables and fruit that are fresh and sweet or sour in taste and protect yin: millet, lemon, orange, mandarin, grapefruit, pear, white mulberry, mango. Choose substances that moisturize dryness, such as honey, acidic and neutral foods such as strawberries, cheese, butter, grapes, pineapple, and medlar. Avoid bitter, spicy, and hot foods that dry out the body.

YIN DEFICIENCY CONSTITUTION:

characterized by symptoms of empty heat: intolerance to heat, restlessness, red cheeks, night sweats, tendency to constipation. There is a predisposition to hypertension, diabetes, heart disease, and a tendency to blood stagnation. Red tongue with little or no coating. Circulation should be promoted with foods that stimulate without drying, such as turnips and radishes, chard, eggplant, tomatoes, mushrooms, black soybeans, saffron, and turmeric. Sweet, fresh, cold foods that produce fluids and nourish yin are useful: especially fresh fruit (apples, pineapples, mangoes, pomegranates, pears, lemons) and vegetables grown in water (such as watercress and water chestnuts), tomatoes, asparagus, white beans, peas, green beans, tofu, and diascorea; horse and rabbit meat, oysters, clams, cuttlefish, crab, chicken and duck eggs, milk, and cheese. Toucha tea is also beneficial. Avoid spices, pepper, chili peppers, alcohol, coffee, tobacco, cured meats, and excessive salt, which dry out and consume fluids and yin. However, do not overindulge in foods that are too cold or raw.

To conclude the discussion on diet and nutrition, we will analyze the recommendations based on the seasons of the year and... the seasons of man, because these must also be taken into consideration. Like every life cycle (or annual cycle), each individual has their own spring (childhood), summer (adolescence), fourth season (maturity), autumn (old age), and winter (senility), each with its own energy level and different balances between the San Bao, so it is advisable to nourish the most deficient elements judiciously.

Seasons: nutrition must also be in tune with the place and season.

SPRING:

it is necessary to regulate the liver; it is advisable to get up early, go for walks, and be aware of the tendency towards irritability as yang energy grows. Sweet and sour foods calm liver tension. The liver suffers from acute sweetness (licorice), green vegetables pacify it. Transform the moisture accumulated in winter, aid digestion with ginger, do not overeat. Green vegetables, wild herbs, spring onions, mulberry leaf infusions, peppermint, chrysanthemum flowers, fresh mushrooms, leeks, garlic.

SUMMER:

It is necessary to purify the heart. Soak up the morning sun. Eat fresher, more raw foods, but remember that digestion is a warm process, so do not flood or freeze. Purify heat with "white tiger decoction," i.e., watermelon, which is sweet, nourishing, and purifies heat with urine. Green tea should be lukewarm, not cold, as it is naturally cool; when iced, it loses its ability to transform phlegm and actually produces it. Green soybeans in soup with lotus seeds. Fresh eggplant, daikon, limit fats, limit meat, especially grilled meat, prefer fish, avoid alcohol.

230

AUTUMN:

In China, this is the dry season, but here it is more variable. If it is still hot, continue with summer foods; if it is dry, protect the yin of the lungs (dry coughs, dry skin). Pears with skin, white mushrooms, white sesame seeds, a little more meat such as neutral and fresh duck until the weather turns cold, then introduce chicken. Persimmons nourish the yin of the lungs and thin phlegm. Avoid hot and drying foods.

WINTER:

It is necessary to support kidney yang, with caution because it cannot be separated from yin. Warmer meats such as mutton, lamb, bone soup (cooked for hours) that penetrate deeply. A little alcohol, soy, legumes, seeds, hazelnuts, walnuts. Avoid raw vegetables and out-of-season , prefer cabbage and savoy cabbage, vegetables fermented with salt (good for the kidneys).

Diet according to the seasons of man

Children:

has specific energetic characteristics that determine his susceptibility to illness but also the speed of change. Remedies, foods, and massage are quickly effective. In early childhood: an immature and weak spleen that easily produces moisture that accumulates in the lungs in the form of mucus (rhinorrhea, otitis, bronchitis) or in the intestines (diarrhea, vomiting). Food and mucus easily become stagnant. The spleen controls the limbs, and until the child has reached maturity, it is unable to control them (important for food choices). Yang hyperactivity, which easily leads to hyperthermia complicated by spasms and convulsions. The predisposition to excess heat manifests itself in behavior that is physiologically lively but can become excessive (hyperkinetic children). Food choices have a significant impact on the heat component (chocolate, animal fats). The diet should be light, with moderate flavor; tonify the spleen and nourish the yin with foods that are neutral in nature and have a bland and moderately sweet flavor. The consumption of well-cooked cereals, little meat, and animal products should prevail; cooked vegetables and fruit without excess (be careful with bananas). Avoid cold foods (ice cream, cold drinks, raw vegetables, too much cheese, fruit juices, fresh juices, antibiotics). They slow down growth by damaging the yang of the spleen and produce moisture; chocolate and other hot foods generate additional heat. Meal times (including breastfeeding) are important. In case of weakened digestion, it can be treated with rice porridge (brown crust in decoction) and lotus flour creams.

In the second and third stages of childhood, the digestive system is mature and children need a lot of nutrition. Excess heat, which is functional for growth, should be treated with sweet, neutral cereals, fresh vegetables, cold foods, fish, chicken (small amounts but frequently), and fruit (preferably whole rather than in juice). If you have digestive difficulties, use sprouted seeds (barley) and hawthorn fruit.

Adolescents:

can digest everything given the great capacity for transformation during this period of life, but it is better for their future not to stress this capacity. Green vegetables, whole foods, meat (including red meat), bone broth, and marrow. Limit the use of sugars and fats if there are signs of heat and humidity, such as acne, which can be treated with herbal teas made from honeysuckle and chrysanthemum flowers, Job's tears, dandelion, and diascorea. In girls with , it is important to nourish and activate the blood with sweet and warm foods, the action of which can be enhanced with Angelica sinensis and Lycium chinensis in infusions or soups, black jujubes, longan, black mushrooms, carrots, and spinach. The uterus must be protected from the cold, especially during this period of menarche, to avoid dysmenorrhea (exposed abdomen, cold baths). Acne can be treated locally by applying a paste of powdered green soybeans and water at night.

Maturity:

physiologically, at 40 years of age, kidney yin is halved and no longer nourishes the liver sufficiently. Diet should be tonifying, avoiding excesses and imbalances that tend to become chronic. Avoid foods that are too hot or too cold, alcohol, fats, and salt. Choose foods carefully based on your constitution and lifestyle. Do not neglect nutrition during the most active period of your life.

Senility:

At this stage of life, our energy levels are the result of our lifestyle habits. There is a physiological decline in yin and yang, which varies in severity depending on our constitution. For women, yin usually declines first, while for men, yang declines first. The reduction in yang affects the spleen: food intake should be reduced and cold foods and foods that are cold in nature and temperature should be avoided. Tonify and warm the body. If there is a yin deficiency (dryness), nourish the kidneys and stomach. Aid digestion and keep the intestines moist (if constipated). Prefer pears, white mushrooms, black soybeans, black sesame seeds, pine nuts, walnuts, lotus seeds, little meat and fat, and avoid excessive salt. Low back pain, which indicates a decline in kidney yang when combined with coldness, pollakiuria, and asthenia, can be improved with: star anise (6g powder) in wine or hot salted water before meals, or with roasted chestnuts (7 per day) or rice soup with pork kidney. Constipation in the elderly can be treated with sweet almonds (15g) and apricots (with the pits and skins removed), cooked in 30g of rice, 30g of sugar, and water until a cream is obtained, to be eaten in the morning and evening.

Menopause:

This is the period of Jing decline, which in women manifests itself with the cessation of menstruation and in men in a less obvious way. It is rarely asymptomatic but is preceded and followed by various disorders resulting from an imbalance between energy and blood, yin and yang. Diet is fundamental and, with the addition of remedies, can correct its evolution. The front heaven cannot be increased and must be supported by the rear heaven, i.e., good digestion. Moderately sweet foods of a neutral nature are preferable, such as cereals at every meal with a small amount of meat or fish, vegetables, and fruit of a balanced nature. Avoid excessive consumption of sugar and industrial sweets, ice cream, raw vegetables, alcohol, spices, and coffee. To meet calcium requirements (osteoporosis), regular consumption of walnuts, almonds, fish cooked for a long time to be eaten with the bones, bone broth, and marrow is recommended. If there is a deficiency of kidney YIN (with empty heat), eat acidic, bitter, salty, and cool foods such as pork meat and marrow, oysters and crab, lotus seeds, grapes, spinach, tomatoes, lettuce, and Chinese cabbage. If the picture is complicated by yang hyperactivity: you can lower the yang (with barley, beef or pork bone broth, celery, asparagus, apples, bananas, lettuce, mint) and calm the mind (longan, jujubes, oysters, rice, wheat, mushrooms). For restlessness, drink a decoction of wheat husks (9g), licorice (6g), and jujubes (5 pieces) for a few days. If there are symptoms of YANG deficiency: use moderately sweet or spicy foods that are warm in nature (mutton, shrimp, chicken, quail, eggs, cherries, chestnuts, peanuts, pine nuts, walnuts).

www.ingramcontent.com/pod-product-compliance
Lightning Source LLC
Chambersburg PA
CBHW052311220526
45472CB00001B/69